"The *MS Workbook* is the most in-depth guide to living well with MS that I have seen yet. The pages are filled with practical, reader-friendly information on everything from cognitive challenges and fatigue, to relapse triggers and unconventional therapies. But it is the checklists, worksheets, exercises, and quizzes that will actively engage readers and empower them to fully incorporate these life-changing strategies."

—*Tammi Robinson Director of Program Services and Outreach The Multiple Sclerosis Foundation*

"This incredibly valuable workbook can help people with MS better understand and cope with their disease. It's an easy-to-follow guide to a better quality of life that includes clear illustrations, checklists, and quizzes devoid of confusing medical lingo. A must-have for patients, it focuses on the challenges (and opportunities) of dealing with MS."

—*Jack Burks, MD, vice president and chief medical officer of the Multiple Sclerosis Association of America*

"I welcome *The MS Workbook* into the library of resources for people living with MS. This comprehensive, user-friendly workbook provides a valuable roadmap for those who are navigating the challenges of MS. Recognizing the potential impact of MS on virtually every aspect of daily life—including the physical, emotional, social, vocational, and spiritual—the authors have assembled for people with MS and their concerned others an array of useful tools for coping, decision-making, and problem-solving."

—*Rosalind Kalb, Ph.D., director of the Professional Resource Center of the National Multiple Sclerosis Society and a clinical psychologist specializing in the care of people with MS and their families*

"Two thumbs way up for *The MS Workbook!* I will recommend this practical, concise, and easy-to-read book to all my c lients with multiple sclerosis. The workbook simplifies difficult to understand but frequently encountered concerns for both the recently diagnosed and those who have been living with multiple sclerosis for years. Examples of topics addressed include stress and mood, employment, health insurance, complimentary and alternative medicine, managing cognitive changes, sexuality and applying for disability insurance. The workbook goes beyond just information sharing and provides numerous worksheets, checklists, and self-assessment tools to promote problem solving and action. The workbook is written with a can-do, take-charge approach, designed to empower those with multiple sclerosis. The workbook's practical advice on living with multiple sclerosis is invaluable and will quickly become the standard resource in the coming years."

—*Daniel E. Rohe Ph.D. ABPP, associate professor of psychology at the Mayo Clinic College of Medicine*

"*The MS Workbook* helps people with MS take control of the challenges presented by chronic illness. This is the first step in resuming important life roles and maintaining a positive quality of life."

—*Richard T. Roessler, Ph.D., CRC, university professor in the Department of Rehabilitation, Human Resources, and Communication Disorders in the College of Education and Health Professions at the University of Arkansas and former codirector of the National Multiple Sclerosis Employment Project*

THE MS WORKBOOK

LIVING FULLY WITH MULTIPLE SCLEROSIS

ROBERT T. FRASER, PH.D. • GEORGE H. KRAFT, MD
DAWN M. EHDE, PH.D. • KURT L. JOHNSON, PH.D.

New Harbinger Publications, Inc.

Copyright © 2006 by Robert Fraser, George Kraft, Dawn Ehde, and Kurt Johnson
New Harbinger Publications, Inc.
5674 Shattuck Avenue
Oakland, CA 94609

Cover design by Amy Shoup
Acquired by Spencer Smith and Jess O'Brien
Edited by Kayla Sussell
Text design by Tracy Marie Carlson

Distributed in Canada by Raincoast Books
All Rights Reserved
Printed in the United States of America

Library of Congress Cataloging-in-Publication Data

The MS workbook : living fully with multiple sclerosis / Robert T. Fraser
   ... [et al.].
     p. cm.
   Includes bibliographical references.
   ISBN 1-57224-390-2 (pbk.)
   1. Multiple sclerosis. 2. Multiple sclerosis—Patients—Psychological
aspects. 3. Self-care, Health.   I. Fraser, Robert T.
RC377.M79 2005
362.196'834—dc22
                                        2005029564

New Harbinger Publications' Web site address: www.newharbinger.com

08   07   06

10   9   8   7   6   5   4   3   2   1

First printing

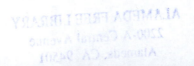

This workbook is dedicated to those of you with MS and your concerned others who, despite the challenges presented by this disability, constantly seek new strategies to counter these difficulties with optimistic fervor.

Contents

CHAPTER 1

Optimizing Your Medical Management   3

Theodore R. Brown, MD, MPH, MS Hub, Seattle, Wa; Barbara Severson, ARNP[1]; George H. Kraft, MD[1]

CHAPTER 2

Getting Things Done: Managing Your Time and Energy   23

Kathryn M. Yorkston, Ph.D, BC-NCD[1]; Estelle R. Klasner, Ph.D[1]; Brian J. Dudgeon, Ph.D, OTR[1]

CHAPTER 3

Perspectives on Psychotherapy   35

Dawn M. Ehde, Ph.D[1]

CHAPTER 4

Health-Promoting Behaviors   47

Charles H. Bombardier, Ph.D

CHAPTER 5

Managing Depression, Anxiety, and Your Emotional Challenges   65

Dawn M. Ehde, Ph.D[1]; Charles H. Bombardier, Ph.D

CHAPTER 15

Tapping Available Community Resources

David C. Clemmons, Ph.D, C.R.C.[1]; Nancy J. Holland, Ed.D. RN National Multiple Sclerosis Society, New York, New York

APPENDIX A

Work Experience Survey

APPENDIX B

U.S. Department of Labor Employment Standards

APPENDIX C

Employer Incentives for Hiring a Worker with a Disability

APPENDIX D-1

Important Federal Regulations Relating to Multiple Sclerosis and Claims for Disability Benefits from the Social Security Administration

APPENDIX D-2

General Considerations for Medical Reports in a Social Security Claim

APPENDIX D-3

The Daily Activity Questionnaire

APPENDIX D-4

Document the Impact of Your Multiple Sclerosis with Diary and Worksheets

Resources

References

[1] All of these authors/coauthors are faculty members of the University of Washington Multiple Sclerosis Rehabilitation Research and Training Center sponsored by the National Institute of Disability and Rehabilitation Research (grant No. H133B031129).

Foreword

Although there has been considerable buzz about "empowerment" and "self-management" in multiple sclerosis (MS), too little of a concrete nature has been done to advance these laudable goals. Successful self-management demands three elements: an attitude of independence; comprehensive, accurate information; and strategies to utilize that information in an active way. There are some excellent consumer-oriented publications on MS and much useful information is available from the National Multiple Sclerosis Society. However, while many sources of MS information exist, the present volume goes one step further.

In addition to offering the reader a wealth of useful information, the authors have provided a number of tools to help readers make the most effective use of that information. Numerous checklists and worksheets will help the person with MS to make the transition from passive reader to active manager. As a result, the pages of this book come alive with myriad possibilities for change and better management of MS.

Starting with an in-depth discussion of each topic, the authors then guide the reader through various strategies to address the issues that arise with each new topic. Citations to the latest scientific and clinical literature will help the person with MS to pursue those topics in greater depth. In addition, interactive exercises, resource lists, and the many tools contained in several appendices make this volume the most comprehensive guide to self-management of MS to appear to date.

By reading this book and using the tools it offers, the person with MS will be well-equipped to partner with health care providers, family, friends, employers, and others to successfully manage MS and its impact on daily life. So, sharpen your pencil, find a comfortable chair, and get ready to take charge of your MS.

—Nicholas G. LaRocca, Ph.D.
Director, Health Care Delivery and Policy Research Program at
the National Multiple Sclerosis Society
New York, NY

Acknowledgments

The editors would like to thank all of the chapter contributors to the workbook both internally within the University of Washington Multiple Sclerosis Rehabilitation Research and Training Center and, externally, Maureen Manley, Peter McKee, Alan Wittenburg, and Drs. Bowling, Foley, Holland, and Rumrill. These are very busy people who had the dedication and took the time to make this workbook a reality. Ms. Kai Martin is thanked profusely for all her hard work and attention to detail in preparing the manuscript. We appreciate Chris Shwartzenburg for his assistance with references and research. We would particularly like to acknowledge our service consumers with MS who helped us through focus groups and other input on critical emphases for this workbook. Ms. Carmen Orso and Mrs. Brenda Vander Lugt were especially helpful in reviewing different aspects of the workbook. If this text is of value to others with MS, it is largely because of these committed individuals.

Finally, we would like to recognize both our publisher, New Harbinger Publications, and our grant sponsor, the National Institute of Disability and Rehabilitation Research-OSERS (U.S. Department of Education, grant number H133B031129). Dr. Matthew McKay and staff at New Harbinger reached out to us for this project and we could not have completed it without the New Harbinger editorial staff: Spencer Smith, Heather Mitchener, Jess O'Brien, and the most detailed work by Kayla Sussell.

All net proceeds from the sale of the workbook, since grant sponsored, will be utilized for further training activities and material dissemination by the University of Washington MS Rehabilitation Research and Training Center.

Introduction

This book began at a psychosocial symposium presented by the faculty members of the University of Washington Rehabilitation Research and Training Center at the American Psychological Association Annual Convention in San Francisco in 1998. Dr. Matthew McKay, the publisher of New Harbinger Publications, was in the audience and it was his idea to develop a workbook that would truly help the person with MS to better cope with the illness from both medical and psychosocial perspectives. As chiefly academics, the book's contributors benefited from our dynamic interchanges with New Harbinger's staff in order to translate our research and other clinical expertise into a format that would be both easily understood and useful to readers. We hope that we were successful in our efforts.

In addition to important information for people with MS, each chapter has worksheets, quizzes, planning exercises, and other materials that can become the basis for your personal planning and coping efforts. You may believe that your specific concerns are addressed only in a few chapters, but we encourage you to read through at least all of the headings in other chapters because you may be pleasantly surprised by the available information, helpful tips, and other materials that you will find.

For example, you may be very satisfied with your medical care, but you may not be aware of some of the travel tips relating to your disability that are outlined in chapter 1. Your job may not be threatened, but you may be unaware of a number of accommodation approaches that could make your life much easier in the workplace, as found in chapter 8.

In sum, we certainly encourage you to spend more time with the chapters that are concerned with life areas of critical concern for you, but other chapters will also merit your review. You can use the worksheets and checklists directly within the chapters and you can copy them as the need arises when you are working on multiple symptoms management and other more extensive concerns. In any case, we commend you on your efforts to better cope with your disability's symptoms, and we truly hope that this workbook will be just one more step in your journey of learning how to live a complete and full life with your disability.

—The Editors

CHAPTER I

Optimizing Your Medical Management

Theodore R. Brown, MD, MPH

Barbara Severson, ARNP, and George H. Kraft, MD

Multiple sclerosis is a complex disability. The two goals of this chapter are for you to understand your disability and gain a wider perspective on ways to manage it. You do have choices in getting a better handle on your multiple sclerosis (MS).

THE PREVALENCE OF MULTIPLE SCLEROSIS

As a person with multiple sclerosis, you are certainly aware of your own situation, but it may be helpful to know that you are not alone. In Western countries, where MS afflicts one in 1,000 people, it is the leading nontraumatic cause of neurological disability in young adults (LaRocca 2005). MS is not new and has probably existed for hundreds or even thousands of years. Perhaps the first case to have been described was that of St. Lidwina of Schiedam (1380–1433), although Charcot in France is credited with having described and established MS as a unique disease in 1877.

MS affects millions worldwide and approximately 400,000 Americans (Rosenberg 2005). Caucasians, especially those of Northern European heritage, have higher rates than other races (Rosenberg 2005). MS is rare in equatorial areas of the world and more frequent at higher latitudes both north and south of the equator (Guarnaccio and Booss 2005). This geographic gradient is also found within the U.S., where the states of Vermont and Washington have the highest prevalence rates in the country (Kurtzke 2005).

Children may be affected by MS, but the age of onset is usually between ages fifteen to fifty (Rosenberg 2005). The peak age of onset for the most common type of MS, the type called "relapsing-remitting MS," is in the late twenties (Kraft and Cui 2004). Women are affected more than twice as often as men, a gender predilection that is found in a host of other autoimmune diseases, including rheumatoid arthritis, lupus, and Graves' disease (Rosenberg 2005).

In the United States, MS appears to be more common in upper socioeconomic groups (Kraft and Taylor 1998). This may be related to genetic factors, unidentified environmental factors that are more common in well-to-do households, or due to the better access to medical care that affluent people have.

WHAT CAUSES MS?

The short but unsatisfying answer to the question above is "we don't know." Certainly, genetics play a part in determining who gets the disease. The risk of a daughter of someone with MS also acquiring the disease is about 3 percent—that's more than tenfold higher than the risk for the general population (Hensiek, Roxburgh, and Compston 2003). The risk for an identical twin is about 30 percent (Guarnaccio and Booss 2005). Although this fact demonstrates the hereditability of MS, it also indicates that MS is not purely genetic, or the risk for an identical twin of someone with MS would be about 100 percent.

If you have MS, it is a combination of genes, not one single gene, that predisposes you to getting the disease. The HLA gene group, used to match organ donors with recipients, is where some of the genes linked to MS have been found. These genes help the immune system to distinguish self from nonself. The protein products of these genes may set the stage for an immune response against the brain in MS in much the same way that they can trigger rejection of a mismatched donor organ.

Epidemiological data suggests that MS is caused or triggered by an environmental factor in people who are genetically susceptible. Whatever the trigger, it appears that it occurs years before the onset of MS (Kurtzke and Wallin 2000). We still have a long way to go before the environmental factors are well understood. For example, we've learned that smoking doubles the risk of getting MS, but we haven't got a clue yet whether it is a chemical (or chemicals) in the tobacco smoke or something else in the smokers' environment, such as lighter fluid, that may contribute to the disease.

Great efforts have been made to uncover just what in the environment might be causing MS. It could be a virus, such as the Epstein-Barr virus, but many investigations of many different viruses have been inconclusive. Vaccinations, bacterial infections, head injury and trauma, stress, cold climate, vitamin deficiency, sunlight deficiency, exposure to dogs, processed foods, and fat have all been studied, but the jury is still out as to what specific factors in the environment cause MS. We do know with some certainty that claims of toxins, dental amalgams, or food substitutes causing MS are baseless (Bowling 2001).

HOW DOES YOUR IMMUNE SYSTEM RELATE TO YOUR MS?

The immune system is vital to protecting humankind against an environment teeming with bacteria, viruses, and other pathogens (what your mother might call "germs"). It even protects us against cancer. In MS, the immune system conducts what could euphemistically be called "friendly fire." What this means is the immune response is misdirected against elements of our own bodies, specifically the central nervous system (CNS), which is composed of the brain, brain stem, and spinal cord. Nerves running from the spine out to the limbs and muscles are not directly affected by MS.

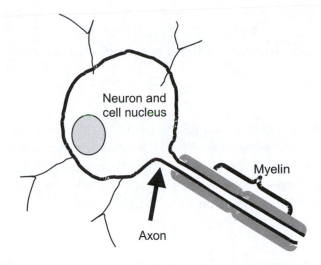

Neuron and
cell nucleus

Myelin

Axon

Figure 1.1: Myelin, the target of the attack.

Through very complex signaling mechanisms, white blood cells known as *T cells* ("T" because they mature in the thymus gland in the chest) become sensitized against submicroscopic particles. Once activated in the blood, they migrate across the blood-brain barrier into the brain. Once inside the nervous tissue, these white blood cells induce an immune reaction (inflammation) against *myelin*, which is a substance composed of fat and protein that functions as insulating material for nerves. The resulting myelin damage is called *demyelination*.

Nerve branches (called *axons*) and the cell bodies of neurons are also damaged as bystanders in this inflammatory process. The inflammation is usually patchy. Each patch is referred to as a *lesion*; lesions usually vary in diameter from the size of a peppercorn (3 mm) to the size of a nickel (2 cm).

Once a new lesion appears on your brain MRI (magnetic resonance image), it usually stays there permanently. This doesn't necessarily mean that it is a lost cause. The brain has repair mechanisms to restore myelin, a process called *remyelination*. Partial or complete remyelination occurs in about half of all MS lesions. Even when MS lesions are completely remyelinated, however, the myelin is thin and doesn't function perfectly. To keep it simple, let's remember that "demyelination" is bad and "remyelination" is good.

THE FOUR TYPES OF MS

Multiple sclerosis is a *heterogeneous disease*, which means that it can affect you in many different ways. There are four basic types of MS, although there are several other rare variations of MS-related disease. If you have MS, it usually begins with an attack of neurological symptoms that subside partly or completely in a few weeks or months. Such attacks are called "exacerbations" or "relapses."

1. If you have the most common type of MS, known as *relapsing-remitting MS (RRMS)*, you will have sporadic exacerbations, at an average rate of about once every seventeen months, but you are neurologically stable between exacerbations.

2. Over a few decades, most people with RRMS (about two-thirds) progress to a second type of MS, known as *secondary-progressive MS (SPMS)*. Rather than having a stable baseline punctuated by exacerbations, people with SPMS have a gradual, progressive decline in function while exacerbations become less frequent. The only way to get to SPMS is by first having passed through RRMS. This is a definitely difficult road to hoe, but new medications are helping us slow this progression.

3. About 10 percent of people with MS begin with progressive disease from the beginning without any sharp exacerbations or remissions. You are then said to have *primary-progressive MS (PPMS)*. With PPMS, you tend to be older at diagnosis than people with RRMS and the ratio of females to males is more equal.

4. The fourth type, *progressive-relapsing MS*, is rare; it shows progression from the beginning along with relapses.

Pathological analysis of brain specimens also has found four basic patterns of the disease that involve differences in immunological activity and cell death. These patterns, however, don't match up with the four clinical types of MS that the patients carried.

There is speculation that MS ultimately may prove to be a syndrome caused by a small number of separate diseases that may require different treatments. Incidentally, the only way to do such pathological analysis is by having a brain biopsy or an autopsy. Obviously, neither of these options is very appealing.

THE MEDICAL DIAGNOSIS OF MS

Medical diagnosis depends on the nature of the disease. If a disease is hereditary, it can now be diagnosed by testing the patient's DNA for the specific genetic marker of the disease. Infectious diseases are diagnosed by identifying the invasive organism with a microscope by isolating it *in vitro* (outside the body and in an artificial environment), or by finding antibodies produced by the host's body to fight against the organism within the host's tissues or fluids.

For all immunological diseases including MS, however, there is no genetic, bacterial, or viral test that can make the diagnosis. Immune disorder diseases are generally diagnosed by criteria that include clinical information (physical examination and symptom history) and laboratory findings (self-antibody tests and pathology results).

In MS, magnetic resonance imaging (MRI) of the brain and spinal cord and electrical tests of nerve pathways also can help in establishing the diagnosis. When there is uncertainty about the diagnosis of MS, a lumbar puncture (also called an "LP" or "spinal tap") may help to make or break the diagnosis by allowing inspection of the cerebrospinal fluid.

The Criteria Used to Diagnose MS

There are detailed criteria for diagnosing MS, the current standard of which is called the McDonald Criteria (McDonald et al. 2001). Here, we will provide a simplified explanation. The basic concept is that MS requires multiple abnormalities (that's why it's called "multiple" sclerosis) and that these abnormalities must involve the central nervous system. The most frequent initial abnormalities are, in descending order: (1) sensory (numbness and tingling of a limb or the face); (2) visual (loss or alteration of vision in one eye); (3) weakness and walking difficulty; (4) incoordination (an inability to coordinate muscular movements); (5) double vision; (6) vertigo; (7) bladder, bowel, or sexual dysfunction; (8) cognitive problems. These multiple abnormalities must occur in a pattern that fits the formula.

How the Diagnosis Is Applied

There is a very standard procedure in diagnosing MS that may be helpful for you to understand. Making the MS diagnosis boils down to the following formula: SIT + SIS + NBE. SIT stands for "Separation In Time." The time between the onset of two abnormalities must be more than thirty days. This is an arbitrary cutoff point that was chosen to aid in diagnosis. SIS stands for "Separation In Space." This means the abnormalities must be at different sites of the CNS. NBE stands for "No Better Explanation." This means corroborating tests are consistent with MS (e.g., MRI shows lesions only in the white matter of the brain, lumbar puncture shows elevated or specific immune globulins in the cerebrospinal fluid compared with the serum), and tests for alternative diagnoses (e.g., viral infection) are negative.

A Short Checklist for a Diagnosis of MS

Generally, all three boxes must be checked to make the diagnosis. However, a new lesion on follow-up MRI can be taken as evidence of a second attack to establish the Separation In Time criteria.

- ☐ Two or more neurological symptoms or signs; onset separated by more than thirty days. (Separation In Time [SIT])

- ☐ Abnormalities found in two or more different sites in the central nervous system. (Separation In Space [SIS])

- ☐ Your doctor has considered other possibilities and found no evidence of another cause. (No Better Explanation [NBE])

Worksheet 1, below, will help you better understand the diagnosis process. Why don't you try to answer the following questions before you read the answers that follow.

WORKSHEET 1:   HOW TO APPLY THE FORMULA FOR DIAGNOSIS

A.   Neal had an attack of arm numbness, arm weakness, imbalance, and confusion all starting one after another over a month-long period. The brain MRI shows multiple lesions in the white matter. Tests for diseases other than MS are all negative. Does Neal have MS?

B.   Tammy has had seven attacks of visual changes in the past four years. Her MRIs and evoked potential tests show lesions at both optic nerves, but no other sites in the central nervous system. Does Tammy have MS?

C.   Mary has kidney disease due to *vasculitis* (inflammation of blood vessels). She developed paraplegia from a spinal cord lesion. Four months later, she noticed double vision when she looked down or to one side. Her MRIs show one lesion in the spinal cord and another in the midbrain. Does Mary have MS?

D.   Rod has never had an "attack" of symptoms. Over five years, he has gradually noticed weakness and spasticity in his legs, bladder urgency, memory and concentration problems that interfere with his job, and fatigue that is much worse in hot weather. His MRIs show multiple lesions in the brain and spinal cord, and lumbar puncture results are positive for the changes seen in MS. There is no family history or other findings to suggest another disease. Does Rod have MS?

Answers

A.   Neal has the SIS and the NBE, but he doesn't have the SIT, because all of these symptoms occurred within one month. He cannot be diagnosed with MS until he suffers another attack. His doctors might advise treatment for MS anyway, because he is at high risk for developing the disease.

B.   Tammy cannot be diagnosed with MS because she doesn't have the SIS. Her diagnosis of MS will have to wait until she develops an abnormality other than visual loss. In the meantime, she will be treated for recurrent optic neuritis.

C.   Mary has both SIT and SIS. However, she has vasculitis that can damage the central nervous system in a way similar to MS. Her diagnosis cannot be MS, because she fails the NBE clause.

D.   Even though Rod has not had MS attacks, he still has evidence of SIT, SIS, and NBE. He could be diagnosed with primary-progressive MS.

YOUR PROGNOSIS AS A PERSON WITH MS

Over the first two years, the course of your MS predicts how you will do in the long run. If you have multiple attacks every year and significant disability by five years, you are probably not going to do as well as someone who experiences two attacks and no disability after five years. Men tend to have a worse prognosis than women. And those whose disease starts after the age of forty tend to do worse than those with earlier onset (Kraft et al. 1981).

Studies of large numbers of patients have provided a rough estimate of what can be expected. Your mild disability could mean marked involvement of one aspect of the CNS, such as sharply decreased touch sensitivity or pain sensation in one limb, or mild abnormalities in several areas of the CNS. The median time until a cane may be required is twenty years, and median time for wheelchair assistance is approximately thirty years (Pittock et al. 2000).

Based on clinical neuropsychological assessments, approximately 45 to 65 percent of individuals with MS exhibit some form of cognitive limitation (Rao 1995). These limitations, however, may or may not impair daily living activities or working. Impaired recent memory, slowing of information processing, abstract reasoning, and problem solving are the most frequent cognitive problems. (See chapter 10 for information about having your potential concerns assessed.)

With time, people with MS tend to acquire more brain lesions. As the brain lesions seen on the MRI increase, cognitive problems tend to worsen. Cognitive function does not correlate well with the physical deficits caused by MS. You may physically feel reasonably good, but be losing some ground cognitively. Even the medical community did not understand this well for years. It is, however, important for you to bear in mind that these facts are based on patient data from an era when most people were generally not treated for MS. There is good reason to believe that the prognosis will improve as medical treatment of the disease improves. Early medication intervention is now the rule.

THE RELATIONSHIP BETWEEN RELAPSES AND DISABILITY

Once you have received a diagnosis of MS, all additional attacks are called "relapses." One group of investigators examined all of the existing U.S. clinical and historical MS data sets to test the effect of relapses on the development of disabilities. They found that each relapse carries a 42 percent chance of adding measurable residual impairment (such as an abnormal sign on physical examination) (Lubin, Baier, and Cutter 2003).

Abnormalities that persist for three months postrelapse usually become permanent. In contrast, French investigators reported that relapse rates predict the development of new disability only up to a point of mild permanent disability (Confavreux et al. 2000). At higher levels of disability, relapse rates do not seem to affect the rate of worsening neurological status. Together, these findings suggest that relapses are associated with worsening disability at the early stages of the disease, but not after marked disability has occurred. Therefore, to have an effect on disability, we say again that your treatment should be started early.

UPDATING YOUR KNOWLEDGE OF MEDICATION

We are fortunate to have several MS disease-modifying medications available for your treatment that will slow the progression of the disease. Although none of the drugs stop MS, they are designed to reduce relapse rates, reduce the number of new lesions on MRI scans, and reduce disability, thereby improving the quality of your life. Medication is selected on a case-by-case basis and determined by what is best for you. It is helpful to remember that medication research study results are based on group averages, however, and that individual responses to medication may differ.

The following medication chart reviews important points when you are selecting an MS disease-modifying medication. These points include consideration of your doctor's recommendations, your personal health, readiness to start treatment, personal choices, lifestyle, support system involvement (family and/or close friends), finances, education about MS disease-modifying medications, and responses to treatment.

If the medication you pick doesn't best meet your needs, you will want to talk with your doctor, make medication adjustments as directed, allow enough time to adjust to the revised treatment plan, and reevaluate how you think the medication is working to slow your disease. If you are having problems taking the medication or you don't like how it makes you feel, let your doctor and nurse know that. They want you to be successful in whatever treatment you choose.

Multiple sclerosis disease-modifying medications are to be taken for a lifetime unless a cure for MS is developed. Luckily, there are many research studies in progress that are giving us new information about current treatments that can lead to changes in medication protocols. Achieving the best outcomes is greatly influenced by an open and honest relationship between you and your significant others, and your doctor, nurse, and healthcare team.

In the U.S., there are currently five Food and Drug Administration (FDA) approved medications for MS. These drugs include three forms of recombinant human interferon:

- Interferon beta-1a (Avonex),

- Interferon beta-1a (Rebif), and

- Interferon beta-1b (Betaseron), and

- a synthetic copolymer glatiramer acetate (Copaxone), and

- a chemotherapeutic agent mitoxantrone (Novantrone).

These five drugs have a direct influence on the course of MS and are designed to slow its progression. Interferon beta-1a, interferon beta-1b, glatiramer acetate, and mitoxantrone are approved for relapsing-remitting MS. Mitoxantrone is also effective for secondary-progressive MS.

The following table of medications will enable you to compare the pros and cons of these medications. Although all these drugs have side effects, most people find them manageable. This table may be very worthwhile for you to review, particularly when you are at the point of deciding what your first medication should be. For a more complete review and comparison of these therapies, see Goodin et al. (2002).

Choosing What Is Best for You

Table 1.1: Multiple Sclerosis Disease-Modifying Medications					
Brand-Name	Avonex	Betaseron	Rebif	Copaxone	Novantrone
Generic Name	Interferon beta-1a	Interferon beta-1b	Interferon beta-1a	Glatiramer acetate	Mitoxantrone
Administration	intramuscular injection	subcutaneous injection	subcutaneous injection	subcutaneous injection	intravenous infusion
Pre-filled Syringe	Yes	No	Yes	Yes	No
Automatic Injection Device	No	Yes	Yes	Yes	No
Frequency of Injections	Once a week	Every other day	Monday, Wednesday, Friday	Daily	Once every three months for up to two to three years only
Injection Site Reaction	Rare	Yes	Yes	Yes	No
Injection Site Necrosis (skin breakdown)	No	Possible	Possible	No	No
Flu-like Symptoms	Yes	Yes	Yes	No	No
Panic-like Reaction	No	No	No	Yes	No
Blood Tests	Yes	Yes	Yes	No	Yes
Refrigeration	Yes	No	Yes	Yes	Not applicable
Stop if Pregnant	Yes	Yes	Yes	Yes	Yes
Patient Training Kit	Yes	Yes	Yes	Yes	Yes
Financial Assistance Program	Avonex Access Program 800-456-2255	Betaseron Foundation 800-998-5777	Rebif MS Lifelines 877-447-3243	National Organization for Rare Disorders 203-746-6518	MS Lifelines 877-447-3243
Patient Support Program	Avonex Alliance 800-456-2255	Pathways 800-788-1467	MS Lifelines 877-447-3243	Shared Solution 800-887-8700	MS Lifelines 887-447-3243

Making the Right Medication Choice

If you need to make a medication choice, the following worksheet may be helpful. You may need to take into account all of the items below, including the actual cost to you of the medication, excluding financial assistance from the relevant pharmaceutical company. Now let's use the worksheet.

WORKSHEET 2:   MEDICATION CHOICES

When considering your choice of medication, you need to consider the following:

Item number   **Your notes/Critical observations**

1.   Doctor's recommendation _____

_____

2.   Personal health choices _____

_____

3.   Readiness to start treatment _____

_____

4.   Lifestyle considerations _____

_____

5.   Support concerns _____

_____

6.   My finances _____

_____

7.   Education about medication _____

_____

8.   Response to treatment _____

My top medication choice(s) are: _____

_____

The material on this sheet can easily be discussed with your doctor or simply used as the basis for your final choice.

THE IMPORTANCE OF EARLY TREATMENT

Early treatment with *immunomodulation* (altering your immune system's responses with the use of a variety of agents) is recommended with the aim of reducing relapses and delaying disability. Research suggests the positive effects of MS disease-modifying medications are maximized if they are started soon after the initial diagnosis of MS is made. If you start taking a medication early in the course of your illness, you will respond better than those who begin treatment later. Treatments show a decrease in relapse rates for patients using the interferons, glatiramer acetate, or mitoxantrone (Goodin et al. 2002).

The National Multiple Sclerosis Society (2005, 1) states, "Initiation of therapy with an immuno-modulator is advised as soon as possible following a definite diagnosis of MS with active disease . . ." You may have heard that this is not the case, but today early medication treatment is the "gold standard" in the treatment of MS. The goal of early intervention is based primarily on the fact that inflammation of the CNS (brain and spinal cord), which is characteristic of MS, may lead to irreversible *axon* destruction, sometimes early in the course of the disease. (An axon is a nerve cell extension that usually conducts impulses away from the cell body.) If you can interrupt this process, then more permanent neurological damage may be delayed. Although the MS disease-modifying medications do not reverse damage, they can decrease future damage.

You may believe that you don't have a sufficient number of MS symptoms or haven't had a sufficient number of relapses to justify starting an MS disease-modifying medication. But it is important to know that many people are unaware of the true number of relapses they have had or are still experiencing. One estimate holds that for every relapse you know about, may have had, or are still experiencing, at least five silent relapses or exacerbations have occurred that you don't know about.

IMMUNOMODULATING MEDICATIONS

In this section you'll find up-to-date information on the medications commonly used for treating MS. These include the interferons, Copaxone (glatiramer acetate), and Novantrone (mitoxantrone). These medications have become widely available only in the last decade.

Interferons

Interferons are naturally produced proteins made by different cells of the body, often in response to infection. These molecules interfere with the replication of many viruses. All interferons can cause flu-like symptoms, such as fever, chills, sweating, muscle aches, malaise, fatigue, and headaches. For most people, these flu-like symptoms lessen or disappear with time. To decrease flu-like symptoms, it is suggested you start the interferon at a reduced dose and slowly increase the dosage over several weeks.

An example would be to start the interferon at a quarter-strength dose for one to two weeks, then increase the amount by one-quarter strength dose every one to two weeks, (as tolerated), up to a full-strength dose. Flu-like symptoms can be effectively managed with acetaminophen (Tylenol), aspirin (Bufferin), or ibuprofen (Motrin) taken before and after the injection. For most people, with time, the need for this preventive medication disappears.

To further manage the flu-like symptoms, it is suggested that you take interferon at bedtime to allow yourself time to sleep through the first several hours, during which time the side effects may occur.

Interferons may cause pain or discomfort at the injection site and abnormal blood tests. It is recommended that blood tests be performed before treatment starts and every three to six months during treatment.

Avonex (Interferon Beta-1a)

Avonex became available in 1996. It is designed for relapsing-remitting forms of MS. It reduces the number of relapses or exacerbations the patient experiences. It is given by *intramuscular injection* (into the muscle) once a week. The amount is 30 mcg/6 million IU, per dose. Avonex is available in a prefilled syringe or as either a liquid or powdered form that you can mix. Because Avonex is injected deep into a muscle, rarely will you see any injection site reaction or feel any injection site discomfort. However, since Avonex is an interferon, it may cause flu-like symptoms.

If you are employed, to initially adjust to the medication, you might want to take Avonex on Friday nights because if flu-like symptoms do occur, they will not happen during a workday. It is recommended you choose the most convenient day of the week for yourself. To learn how to administer the injection yourself, it is best to be taught by a qualified doctor or nurse who is knowledgeable about MS. However, if this is not possible, training may be provided by a nurse recommended by the manufacturer of Avonex.

Avonex has demonstrated: (a) a reduction in relapse rate, (b) a slowing in the disability's functional impairing effect, and (c) a reduction in active lesions as shown on an MRI (Jacobs et al. 1996). Note that it may take several months for the Avonex to begin working.

Rebif (Interferon Beta-1a)

Rebif became available in 2002. In the United States, it is the newest interferon for MS. Rebif is nearly identical to Avonex; however, the two medications differ slightly in their manufacturing process and in the preservatives added to the final solution. Rebif is given by *subcutaneous injection* (in the tissue between the skin and muscle). The recommended dose and schedule for Rebif is 44 mcg three times a week. Ideally, you should take the medication the same three days of each week. For example, inject the Rebif every Monday, Wednesday, and Friday. It is also best to take the medication at the same time each day; preferably at bedtime.

Rebif is supplied in a prefilled syringe. It also comes with an automatic injection device that makes giving the injection easier for you. The automatic injection device also causes reduced injection site skin reactions. Because the Rebif is administered into the subcutaneous tissue, localized injection site skin reactions may last several weeks before disappearing. These reactions may be redness, swelling, itching, and pain.

One serious side effect has been reported in a small number of people using Rebif. That is injection site tissue damage or *tissue necrosis* (tissue death). The necrosis may occur at a single injection site or at multiple injection sites. If an injection site becomes very painful, swollen, or looks infected and doesn't heal within a few days, call your doctor.

There is an ongoing debate over the best Interferon beta-1a (Avonex versus Rebif) dosage and whether the higher weekly dose of Rebif results in better health outcomes. Evidence may indicate that the interferon beta formula, dose, and frequency of injection may influence patient outcomes, with the outcomes showing more favorable change toward the more intense schedules of Rebif and Betaseron (see below). Rebif has demonstrated: (a) a reduction in relapse rate and (b) a reduction in progression of the disease and (c) a reduction in new lesions as seen on an MRI. Regular tests to monitor liver and blood counts are recommended.

Betaseron (Interferon Beta-1b)

Betaseron became available in 1993. It is designed for relapsing forms of MS. It reduces the number of relapses or exacerbations a person experiences. It is given by subcutaneous injection, at a dose of 0.25 mg/8 million IU, every other day. You can also use an automatic injection device with Betaseron. Because the medication is administered into the subcutaneous tissue, localized injection site reactions may occur, and they may last several weeks before disappearing. These reactions can be redness, swelling, itching, and pain.

A serious side effect has been reported in a small percentage of people on Betaseron. That is severe skin damage or tissue necrosis at injection sites. The necrosis may occur at a single or multiple injection sites. If one of the injection sites becomes very painful, swollen, or looks infected and doesn't heal within a few days, call your doctor. You will need to rotate injection sites regularly and use correct injection technique to reduce the chance of this problem occurring. If tissue necrosis does occur, notify your doctor immediately.

Because flu-like side effects may occur with Betaseron, take it at bedtime, with acetaminophen (Tylenol), aspirin (Bufferin), or ibuprofen (Motrin). Start the Betaseron at a reduced dose and gradually work up to taking it at full strength over several weeks.

To learn the best injection technique and how to manage the side effects of medication, we recommend again that you receive training from a doctor or nurse who is knowledgeable about MS. If this is not possible, the manufacturer of Betaseron has a nursing staff who will come to your home and provide injection training. While you are on Betaseron, your blood will need to be monitored regularly. Betaseron has demonstrated: (a) a reduction in relapse rate and (b) a reduction in active lesions as seen on an MRI. Note that it may take several months for the Betaseron to start working. Regular tests to monitor liver and blood counts are recommended.

Copaxone (Glatiramer Acetate)

Copaxone became available in 1996. It is designed for relapsing-remitting MS. It is given by subcutaneous injection every day. The dose is 20 mg per day. For the consumer's convenience, Copaxone comes in a prefilled syringe with an automatic injection device.

Copaxone is not an interferon. It is believed to work by activating anti-inflammatory regulatory T cells, which then migrate into the CNS to inhibit local immune reactions.

Compared to interferons, Copaxone has different side effects. With Copaxone, you may experience localized injection site skin reactions that last for a few days. These reactions typically consist of redness, itching, pain, swelling, and a lump under the skin at the injection site(s). These reactions are usually mild and seldom require medical treatment.

Copaxone has sometimes been associated with a wasting of the fat tissue at the injection site. Also, with this medication there is about a 10 percent chance of experiencing an immediate post-injection reaction that feels like a panic reaction. These symptoms consist of flushing (feeling warm and/or redness), sweating, chest pain or tightness, rapid heart rate, anxiety, throat tightness, and trouble breathing. Usually, this reaction is not harmful and it is not associated with a heart attack or an allergic reaction to Copaxone. These symptoms generally occur within minutes after an injection and last for about fifteen to twenty minutes. They go away by themselves without requiring medical treatment.

If you experience this reaction, sit down, try to relax, take some deep breaths, and wait for the symptoms to pass. Because Copaxone does not cause the flu-like symptoms typical of the interferons, it can be taken at any time of the day. However, you may prefer to take the Copaxone at bedtime when you are less hurried and have more time to attend to the injection. You don't need to take blood tests while taking Copaxone.

Copaxone has demonstrated: (a) a reduction in relapse rate, (b) a reduction in time for disability to occur, and (c) a reduction in active lesions as seen on an MRI. It may take several months for the Copaxone to start working.

Taking Immunomodulating Medications: Building a Support System

It is normal to be nervous about starting an injectable medication. Your doctor and nurse will help you through this difficult period. The first injection is the hardest but it does get easier. It's always a good idea to bring someone with you for your first injection training. Two sets of ears and eyes are better than one. A family member or friend, someone who has been through the teaching, can help you with your injections. Most medication side effects are easily managed. Tell your doctor and nurse if you're having problems, especially if you're thinking about stopping the medication. The flu-like side effects of the interferons usually lessen and disappear after several months.

All MS disease-modifying medications are expensive. However, the good news is all of these medications have financial assistance programs. Speak to your doctor's office staff to find out about these programs. Ultimately, you must decide which drug will work best for you, but your doctor and nurse can help you to make this decision.

Checklist 1: Injection Tips Review

The following information will help you with your MS injections, regardless of which medication you choose. If you're using one of the medications previously discussed, please review these concerns carefully by reading the checklist below and asking yourself all of the following questions:

_____ Before I started using MS disease-modifying medication, did I tell my doctor about all the other medications I'm already taking? (This includes prescription, nonprescription, herbal, and other naturopathic medications.)

_____ Do I check the expiration date on the medication? (Do not use it if it has expired.)

_____ Do I allow the medication time to warm up to room temperature before doing the injection? (Cold solution can hurt.)

_____ If I am unable to inject the medication myself, can a family member or friend be taught the injection technique to help me?

_____ Do I wash my hands and clean my skin before every injection to reduce the risk of infection?

_____ Do I briefly ice my skin, before and/or after an injection to reduce injection site pain or discomfort?

_____ Do I cleanse the injection site with alcohol, or another antiseptic solution, before giving the injection?

_____ Do I allow time for the antiseptic solution to dry before giving the injection?

_____ If the antiseptic solution is irritating to my skin, do I use unscented soap instead?

_____ Do I use a dry injection needle? (Do not squirt any medication out of the syringe and onto the needle before giving the injection, because the medication can burn and irritate the skin.)

_____ There may be small air bubbles in the prefilled syringes of some of the MS disease-modifying medications. Do I try to expel the air bubbles from the syringe before injecting? (**Note:** These air bubbles are _not_ harmful and expelling them may put irritating solution on the tip of the needle, which can get on the skin.)

_____ Do I gently swirl (not shake) the medication that comes in the liquid and powdered form that must be mixed?

_____ Do I try to give myself my injection at the same time every day?

_____ Do I unnecessarily pinch the skin for the subcutaneous injections? (Pinching the skin is not necessary and may bruise the site.)

_____ Do I rotate injections to all skin sites and make sure I spread the injections out around a site? (That is, I don't always come down on the same puncture point.)

_____ Do I avoid administering injections into skin that is reddened, bruised, infected, scarred, or hard?

_____ If I have hives, dizziness, severe pain at an injection site, or other abnormal changes with my health, do I tell my doctor and nurse as soon as possible?

_____ If I use Copaxone, do I avoid massaging the injection site until twenty-four hours after the injection?

_____ Do I use an automatic injection device if one is available?

_____ Have I had the automatic injection device adjusted for different injection site locations?

_____ Do I lightly rest the automatic injection device on the skin? (Do not punch the skin with it.)

_____ Do I ever consider reusing needles or syringes? (**Caution:** Injection needles are for one-time use only.)

_____ Have I checked with my local public health department, doctor, nurse, or pharmacist about needle and syringe disposal? (There may be special state and/or local laws for disposing used equipment. Do not throw needles or syringes directly into the garbage or recycling container.)

_____ Do I store my medication, needles, syringes, and needle disposal container out of the reach of children?

Answer the questions below if they are applicable:

_____ Do I ever consider taking MS disease-modifying medication if I am planning on becoming pregnant, or if I am pregnant, or breast-feeding? (**Caution:** Do not use MS disease-modifying medication if planning on becoming pregnant, or you are pregnant, or breast-feeding.)

_____ If I become pregnant while taking an MS medication, I will stop and tell my doctor.

In terms of my medication and injection procedures, I need to remember the following:

_____

_____

_____

NOVANTRONE (MITOXANTRONE): AN IMMUNOSUPPRESSIVE

Novantrone became available for multiple sclerosis in 2000. It is approved for worsening relapsing-remitting MS, secondary-progressive MS, and progressive-relapsing MS. It has been used as a chemotherapy medication for over ten years in the treatment of breast cancer, prostate cancer, lymphomas, and other malignancies. Novantrone is an *immunosuppressive drug,* which means it suppresses the immune system, and disrupts or kills certain cells in the immune system that play a role in destroying myelin and causing lesions in the brain and spinal cord of MS patients. Other drugs for MS (Avonex, Rebif, Betaseron, Copaxone) are not immunosuppressive, they are *immunomodulators,* which means they alter or change immune responses, they do not suppress them.

Novantrone is given by *intravenous infusion* (into a vein) once every three months for approximately two to three years. It is then stopped because of concerns about heart damage. The risk of permanent and irreversible heart damage usually does not occur until the person with MS exceeds the total lifetime maximum dose of 140 mg/m2. The amount of Novantrone given for each intravenous infusion for MS is usually lower than what a cancer patient receives. In any case, your doctor will want to make sure the harmful effects from the Novantrone are avoided, so your heart will be monitored regularly during treatment and you will undergo additional laboratory tests.

The most common side effects of Novantrone are nausea (upset stomach), fatigue, hair thinning, upper respiratory or bladder infections, loss of menstrual periods, and mouth sores. The nausea is usually mild and generally lasts less than forty-eight hours. It can be managed with antinausea medication that is taken before and after each Novantrone treatment. Because Novantrone is a dark blue in color, your urine and the whites of your eyes may turn blue for a short time after each dose.

Tell your doctor immediately if you develop heart problems, such as trouble breathing, swelling in your ankles or legs, or a fast or uneven heartbeat. These problems generally occur if you receive a total lifetime dose of more than ten doses (usually more than 140 mg/m2) of Novantrone. Within the first several weeks after each infusion, Novantrone can increase your chance of getting an infection, so it is wise to report any signs of infection, such as fever, chills, cough, sore throat, and pain or burning with urination. However, isolation during this period is usually not recommended.

Novantrone can cause irregular or loss of menstrual periods and infertility. Women of childbearing age need to discuss this risk of infertility with their doctor and decide whether this medication is right for them. Women who do decide to take Novantrone must use birth control to avoid becoming pregnant. Your doctor should give you a pregnancy test before each dose of Novantrone. Novantrone should not be taken if you are trying to become pregnant, or breast-feeding. If you become pregnant while on Novantrone you need to tell your doctor right away because Novantrone can harm the fetus and cause birth defects. You should not plan on having children while taking Novantrone and for several months after the final treatment ends. Novantrone may also stop sperm production in men.

Before starting Novantrone, tell your doctor if you have any present or past history of: heart disease, cancer chemotherapy, liver disease, problems with your immune system, abnormal blood tests, blood-clotting problems, infections, unusual or unexpected bleeding, allergies or sensitivities, radiation treatment to the chest, or prior treatment with Novantrone. Novantrone affects blood tests and will cause your white blood cell count to go down, which increases your chance of getting an infection. This risk of infection is greatest within one month after each treatment.

The best thing you can do to prevent infection is to practice good hand-washing technique for several weeks after each Novantrone infusion. Novantrone can also cause your blood platelet count to go down, which increases the likelihood of bleeding and bruising. To ensure your safety, the doctor must monitor your blood tests before and after each treatment. Below are reviewed Novantrone concerns.

Checklist 2: Tips Review for Novantrone

In relation to your Novantrone treatments, are you remembering to do the following?

_____ I schedule my Novantrone appointment every three months.

_____ I cancel my Novantrone appointment if I'm sick, and I reschedule it when I'm feeling better.

_____ I tell my doctor or nurse about any problems that I'm having with the Novantrone.

_____ To prevent nausea: (a) I don't eat for a few hours before the infusion. _____ (b) I drink cool, clear, and unsweetened juices. _____ (c) I eat small meals throughout the day. _____

_____ To reduce the chances of my hair thinning after the Novantrone treatments: (a) I use a soft hairbrush and mild shampoo. _____ (b) I don't color or perm my hair. _____ (c) I use low heat when drying my hair. _____

_____ To avoid infection within the first month after every Novantrone infusion: (a) I wash my hands frequently. _____ (b) I avoid people who are sick. _____ (c) I eat a well-balanced diet and drink plenty of fluids. _____ (d) I get adequate rest. _____

_____ I will tell my doctor if I have an uneven or fast heartbeat, chest pain, trouble breathing, or swelling in my hands or feet.

_____ I will not undergo surgery or dental work for several weeks before or after my Novantrone treatment.

_____ I will tell all my doctors and healthcare providers that I am taking Novantrone.

_____ I will not receive injections of live vaccinations while on Novantrone.

The benefits of Novantrone may not be felt until after the third or fourth treatment. This may mean you might not notice a change in your MS symptoms until nine months to a year after beginning treatment. Because Novantrone may cause heart damage during therapy or months to years after therapy ends, you must tell your doctor or nurse if you have any trouble breathing, chest pain or discomfort, or any other health problems.

TRAVELING WITH YOUR MEDICATION

There are a number of issues about traveling with MS disease-modifying medications that are important to remember. The checklist of travel tips below highlights these points and is helpful to review when you go on a trip. Many of you who are newly diagnosed may not be aware of some of these useful tips.

Checklist 3: Travel Tips

_____ I always take my MS disease-modifying medication in my carry-on baggage when I'm traveling.

_____ I always carry my MS disease-modifying medication in its original labeling and packaging.

_____ I bring extra medication with me when I'm traveling because I may wish to stay longer or I may have an unscheduled delay.

_____ I always carry my doctor's business card with his/her name and telephone number.

_____ If I feel ill or have an MS exacerbation when traveling, I watch my symptoms for about twenty-four to forty-eight hours because I may start to feel better. If I think I'm having an exacerbation, I will find medical attention and I may need to go to an emergency room to be seen.

_____ When traveling in the United States, I will carry a list of MS treatment centers located within the country. (This list can be provided by the National Multiple Sclerosis Society.)

Conclusion

Although there is no cure for MS at this time, there are many drugs than can slow down the progression of the disease and improve the quality of your life. The decision of which MS disease-modifying drug to select is ultimately yours. Your doctor, nurse, family, and close friends can help you in selecting the drug that best fits your needs. Hopefully, table 1.1 that compares the different medications will be helpful to you in making your personal choice. If you've forgotten where the table is located, you will find it under the heading Choosing What Is Best for You. It is recommended that you start a drug early to optimally reduce the number and severity of MS exacerbations, the progression of the disease, and the development of disability. Your health care team will work, in partnership with you, toward successful management of your health.

In this chapter, we have discussed only part of the complete medical treatment for MS, i.e., the commonly used medications that directly affect the disease process. There is often more that can be done in your particular case. Medications can be taken to improve various symptoms of the disease, such as fatigue, pain, spasticity, bladder problems, depression, etc. Consult your physician to determine whether any of these types of medication might be helpful to you.

CHAPTER 2

Getting Things Done: Managing Your Time and Energy

Kathryn M. Yorkston, Ph.D., BC-NCD,

Estelle R. Klasner, Ph.D., and Brian J. Dudgeon, Ph.D., OTR

YOUR PERSONAL CHALLENGE

Getting things done involves work. In this chapter, we define *work* in its broadest sense, as an activity that you perform to accomplish something. Your "life's work" can range from taking care of yourself, to cooking a meal for your family, to being a board member of a charitable organization. Work includes doing all of the things in your life that are necessary for survival or have value for you. When you are living with multiple sclerosis (MS), work is often done in the presence of obstacles that may make accomplishing the work difficult.

In this chapter, we outline not only the barriers you may face to participate fully in work, we also describe some ways to deal with these barriers. Finally, we provide suggestions for sources of help to aid you in pursuing the work you wish to accomplish.

BARRIERS TO FULL PARTICIPATION

Before discussing strategies for dealing with difficulties in getting things done, we need to understand the three major difficulties: fatigue, changes in thinking, and stress. Each of these may be a major challenge for you and, in combination, they may create a cycle so vicious that it makes matters even worse. We begin with a description of each barrier and then we will describe how they combine to form a cycle of difficulty that may be greater than the sum of its parts.

FATIGUE

Fatigue is the feeling of lacking the physical and/or mental energy to do the activities you wish to accomplish. If you have MS, fatigue is very common. Almost 80 percent of people with MS experience some level of fatigue and it is the most commonly reported symptom (MacAllister and Krupp 2005). Fatigue is described as being the "worst" symptom by about one-third of those who have MS (Krupp et al. 1988). Fatigue can have a profound influence on your life. What you do, how much you do, and when you can do it can all be disrupted by fatigue. One woman with MS put it simply. She said, "Fatigue dictates my life." The fatigue associated with MS is different from the types of fatigue other people experience (National Multiple Sclerosis Society 2003). Although it may be unpredictable from day to day, it generally occurs on a daily basis and tends to worsen as the day progresses. It is often aggravated by heat and humidity. Finally, fatigue is a challenge because it is invisible to others and may be misinterpreted as depression, a lack of effort, or as just not trying hard enough.

CHANGES IN THINKING

Changes in thinking or memory are also common, occurring in about half of people with MS (LaRocca and Kalb 2005). Like many aspects of MS, changes in thinking vary considerably from person to person due, at least in part, to the location, number, and activity of MS lesions. There is general agreement that changes in thinking are not global; that is, they do not affect all of the functions of the brain but rather target specific processes such as memory and information processing. These changes in thinking can make it difficult for you to do more than one thing at a time or to perform complex tasks when there are time pressures.

At times, fatigue and changes in thinking are difficult to separate from each other. Fatigue can be described in many ways, including weakness, lack of stamina, feeling "spacey," having poor concentration, feeling bored, or just general dissatisfaction. It is important to appreciate the mental aspects of fatigue because often they make thinking clearly more difficult. One man with MS described the mental aspects of fatigue this way: "Fatigue is the cognitive mud that I have to slog through before I can think clearly."

STRESS

Stress is the third in this series of challenges often faced by people with MS. *Stress* can be described as a feeling or sense of uneasiness. It is an internal feeling associated with being anxious or feeling overwhelmed. Situations that previously would not have been stressful for you may become a problem because of diminished capacity for thinking clearly and fatigue. Feeling anxious can be exaggerated by fatigue, changes in thinking, and demanding tasks. You might view stress as clearly undesirable because it is associated with a worsening of symptoms. There are resources are available for achieving more stress-free productivity (see Allen 2001).

It may be helpful for you to consider stress when you evaluate or judge a specific situation and not the situation itself. In other words, any given situation may be viewed as stressful by one person and enjoyable by another. For example, the necessity to juggle many things to do your work may be viewed as either "adding spice to life" or as overwhelming and stressful.

Once you may have thrived on stress related to various activities, but now you may find stress interfering with getting things done. You may become anxious with complex tasks and fearful of failure. The stress may be unpleasant and even emotionally overwhelming. Clearly, cognitive changes and fatigue will influence your evaluation of situations as either stressful or not.

The Vicious Cycle

Fatigue, changes in thinking, and stress can encircle those with MS as shown in figure 2.1. For example, fatigue may bring about difficulty in thinking. The cycle continues, because thinking requires effort and attention and that, in turn, results in more fatigue. A woman with MS described the cycle of changes in thinking and stress this way: "It's kind of like a revolving circle effect, the more stress there is, the more confused I get, and the more confused I get, the more that stresses me." This cycle creates a formidable barrier to getting things done because fatigue, cognitive change, and stress are variable, somewhat unpredictable, and invisible to others. Furthermore, the cycle can be worsened by a variety of external factors like trying to do too much, trying to do too many things at once, demanding situations, or demanding people.

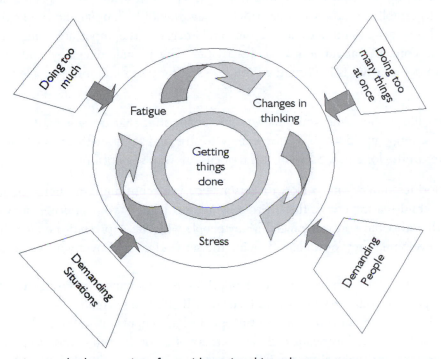

Figure 2.1: The vicious cycle that may interfere with getting things done.

In managing your time and energy, you need to find the right balance in the costs and benefits of getting work done. Your balance can be upset by several factors, including change in the symptoms of MS, daily variability in energy and cognition levels, as well as stressors and other barriers in the environment. Maintaining your balance may require you to initiate and develop a series of strategies with the resources available to you. In the next section, people with MS describe how constructing their sets of strategies enables them to participate fully in life.

DEVELOP YOUR OWN STRATEGIES TO DEAL WITH MS

Many factors make each person with MS unique. These include the set of symptoms that you experience, how these symptoms vary from day to day and over time, the activities you value, and your daily life situations. Although healthcare providers and family members may be well-informed, only you—the person with MS—can truly know about your own experiences. For that reason, only you can decide on the best strategies for yourself.

Over the past five years, we've talked with many people who have MS about what it's like to live with this condition (Johnson et al. 2004; Yorkston et al. 2003). We call the approach to developing strategies these people told us about by the acronym PACE. This provides an easy way to remember the four most important steps: Priorities, Awareness, Constructing your strategies, and Evaluation. The following section provides a step-by-step exercise to help you develop strategies that will work for you.

Priorities

Let's begin with priorities. A *priority* is something you give attention to or focus on before anything else that may be competing for your time or attention. It is what you value. Many people described how MS required them to establish a new set of priorities, a new way of looking at the things they did every day. They described how essential it is to devote time and energy to the important things that you value while reducing your concerns about less valued activities. Given limited energy and resources, it is important for you to define what is important to you, to set priorities. One of the people we interviewed put it this way:

> You learn that life is short and you quit worrying about stuff that doesn't matter. You only have so much energy and don't have the energy to fuss and fiddle with things that are not going to matter in the long run. So you learn to focus on what's important.

Note that priorities differ from person to person. For you, continuing a cherished job may be a priority; for others, child-rearing comes first. If your symptoms worsen, your priorities may change. You need to get in touch with what you value most. Many people with MS expressed the idea that they need to be in charge of developing their own plans. Having the sense of control over your life decisions is very important.

Now it's time for you to figure out what your priorities are. It's important to figure this out so you will know on which parts of your life you want to focus your limited energy and time.

Worksheet 3 lists the five domains that most people feel are important to them. The first domain is called Taking Care of Yourself. This might include a variety of activities you choose to promote for your physical, psychological, or spiritual well-being. Getting adequate exercise, enough rest, and good nutrition might belong to this domain along with other matters like reducing your feelings of stress.

The second domain is Family and Household. This might include your priorities related to the management of your household and the people who live in it. The third domain is Leisure or Discretionary Activities that you enjoy. The fourth is your Career. This may involve paid or unpaid employment or schooling. The final domain is Taking Part in Your Community and it may involve priorities that relate, for example, to the roles you choose to play in your community organizations.

Instructions for Worksheet 3

Try to list two activities you believe are your priorities in each domain. Priorities must be specific, otherwise they will seem unachievable. For example, the priority to "get a good job" is too vague and needs to be more specific. What does "good" mean to you? Does it mean flexible hours, a brief commute, great benefits, or friendly coworkers? Carefully defining your priorities increases the likelihood that you will be able to accomplish them. Then, having met your priorities, you can set new ones. It's okay to start with general priorities so long as you define your terms to make the priority specific, for example, what do you mean by "good" in the priority "getting a good job."

After you've listed your two priorities for each domain, pick the one that is most important to you in each domain. After you do this, pick the domain and its top priority that you want to work on first. It is important to not allow yourself to be overwhelmed by trying to work on too many priorities at once.

WORKSHEET 3:   PRIORITIES

Taking care of yourself: _____

_____

_____

Family and household: _____

_____

Leisure or discretionary activities: _____

_____

Career: _____

_____

Taking part in your community: _____

_____

Awareness

After you've thought about your priorities, you need to become aware of potential barriers to getting things done and the resources you have to get around those barriers. The people we interviewed described a number of factors (or triggers) that caused them to change how they did things. Sometimes the factors were internal and associated with the symptoms of MS, for example, fatigue or changes in thinking. Other factors were associated with the environment and the stresses present in certain situations. For example, a first-grade teacher described how the classroom situation was stressful to her because it required her to pay attention to so many things at one time. She said about her job: "I think it's just overload in a job like this when you must deal with twenty-five first graders and the demands of the day, that sometimes little things would get lost or that you would become forgetful."

Certain internal symptoms or environmental triggers will signal to you that change is needed. The people we interviewed also described the need for vigilance or awareness of the factors that signal the need to change how they handled their affairs. They appeared to monitor their potential triggers very carefully. For example, one woman said, "You have to listen to your body because if you don't listen to your body, you are absolutely going against the current." Another woman had developed a daily self-monitoring routine by doing a crossword puzzle in order to "take inventory." She described it like this:

> The crossword puzzle gives me three kinds of information. One, how's the fine motor control? Are my tremors bad today? Two, how's my cognition? Can I find the words that I'm after? And three, how's my strength and endurance? Do I have the energy to finish the puzzle today?

The degree of awareness you cultivate will give you information about how things are going; it involves being alert for and anticipating potential problems. For you to function at your best, you need to stay vigilant to the clues that changes are needed.

To achieve your priority goals, or to accomplish anything, you must learn about the resources available to you when you need to get the work done. For example, one woman described how she was always "looking for solutions." She had the time and energy to maintain her job outside the home, but only if she hires someone else to clean her house. In addition to providing her with the satisfaction of her work and with social contacts, keeping her job gave her the financial resources to hire the help she needed to maintain her household.

Finding solutions means selecting from the resources available to you. If your resources are limited, you may need to be creative. For example, can a high school or college student clean your house, run errands, shop, or do the other chores that you find difficult or tedious? If you have little money, you might barter to get the help you need (do some computer work for someone, provide a free room in your house, etc.). You can identify what you have to offer to get the critical help that you need.

Now let's continue the work you started when you listed your priorities. In worksheet 4, write down the specific priority that you've selected as your first goal. Then think about barriers that prevent you from accomplishing that goal and write them down. Finally, think about the resources you have that may help you to get around those barriers. Remember to be creative and get help in identifying your resources if that seems necessary.

WORKSHEET 4:   AWARENESS AND CONSTRUCTION OF STRATEGIES

What Priority Are You Working On? _____

Barriers to getting it done: _____

_____

Resources you have: _____

_____

Strategies you might use: _____

_____

Constructing Your Strategies

Many people we interviewed described a process where they began doing things in different ways. One man said, "MS doesn't really affect what I do. Rather, it affects how I do it." Changing how things get done involves constructing and employing a personal set of strategies. This is a process of combining elements in order to accomplish a specific task. In other words, use your strengths and resources to do things. Table 2.1 below shows examples of a number of strategies developed by people with MS along with the factors that triggered their use of these strategies. For example, one woman said that she always takes extensive notes during business meetings because she becomes easily fatigued at long meetings. She commented, "I usually write a lot of notes so that a little bit later, when I have more energy and I'm able to think more clearly, I can review them. Writing things down also helps me think more clearly too."

Table 2.1: A Description of Selected Strategies		
The Strategy	**Benefit of the Strategy**	**Cost of the Strategy**
Take notes during business meetings	Increased attention during meetings and good review of ideas afterward when energy level is higher	Don't participate as actively in the meetings
Begin work at 5 A.M. and leave by early afternoon	Important work done without distractions and when not fatigued	Need to negotiate with supervisors about my work schedule
Midday rest breaks at work in private quiet room	Reduced fatigue and increased concentration	Social isolation from fellow employees during break time
Household organization, e.g., cleaning products always in appropriate locations	Reduced energy expended in finding and gathering supplies before doing household tasks	Others in household must help maintain organization
Desk and parking place reassignment to minimize walking distances	Decreased fatigue	Need to negotiate with employer
Desk clear except for appropriate paperwork	Can concentrate on one thing at a time	Time spent in shifting materials for each task
Making a daily to-do list	Priority tasks were accomplished, reduced the stress of trying to remember everything	Time to construct the listings; appreciating how many things could not be accomplished

Here's an example of a strategy used to compensate for cognitive changes. One woman keeps her desk at work "really neat" with only the papers relating to the task at hand on her desktop. She reported that this prevented her from "getting sidetracked."

Other strategies involve organizational techniques for completing household work. One person we talked to kept a very orderly home. She spoke about her need for order:

> I can't be scattered. Things have to have a place. If I want to go get the furniture polish for cleaning my woodwork, I have to know it's there. I don't want to walk to the hall closet and then discover that it's just not there. That wastes too much energy!

Now let's continue the work you started earlier. Go back to the priority you chose to work on. In worksheet 4, you listed some barriers and also some resources to get around those barriers. Now, we would like you to brainstorm some ways that might help you to accomplish your priorities. While you are doing this, keep two things in mind. First, there are no "wrong" answers. Just come up with anything you can think of as a way to achieve your goal and write it down. Second, keep your barriers and resources in mind and while you are strategizing, think of ways that these barriers may be overcome. If you get stuck, ask for help from a resourceful friend or your significant other.

Evaluating Your Strategies

The last important step to take when developing strategies is for you to evaluate them. Periodically, people with MS need to ask themselves this question: Does this strategy still work for me? You can evaluate your strategies by weighing their costs and benefits (as in table 2.1). For example, an elementary school teacher needs to take rest breaks during her teaching day. She uses a quiet room away from the other teachers' break room where she can relax in a recliner. Although this rest break is both beneficial and necessary, she knows it also has a cost; she commented, "It is rather isolating as well as good for my health."

In this particular case, the benefits outweigh the cost and she continues the practice. For some people, however, the value of their strategies may change over time. Some strategies may be very effective in some situations but less so in others. For these reasons, your evaluation process is important when making decisions about when, where, and with whom to use your strategies.

Once you've employed some of the strategies you thought up, it's essential that you go back and do a final review. This will give you the opportunity to see what helped and what didn't work, and to try out other strategies that might work better.

Use worksheet 5, below, to list the benefits and costs of a strategy you are using. After doing the work, and thinking about this, rate both the benefits and costs of the strategy. These ratings will help you decide whether to continue using these strategies or if you need to modify them.

If a strategy doesn't work for you, go back and try another. Brainstorming with some other people may be a good way to figure out how to make certain strategies work better for you or how to create new ones.

WORKSHEET 5:   EVALUATING YOUR STRATEGIES

What is your strategy? _____

_____

List some ways that it is helpful: _____

_____

_____

Check the appropriate box to determine how helpful this strategy is:

	Very helpful	Helpful	Helps some	Neutral	Not helpful
This strategy is:					

Now, list some of the costs of using this strategy: _____

_____

_____

Check the appropriate box to determine how costly this strategy is:

	Has no costs	Has few costs	Is neutral	Has some costs	Has high costs
This strategy:					

What is your next step?

Continue to use the strategy, or

Modify the strategy in the following way: _____

_____

Or, try the following new strategy: _____

_____

WHERE TO GET HELP

In this final section of the chapter, we will outline some general tips and resources for developing a plan that will work for you. Table 2.2 is a checklist of questions to ask yourself, along with suggestions for the appropriate resources for finding help.

Table 2.2: Identify Sources of Help to Manage Your Time and Energy		
Question	Why your answer is important	Where to get the help you need
Are you exercising regularly?	It improves your fitness and helps you feel less tired	Consult a physical therapist
Do you eat the right foods?	The right diet can help keep your energy high	Consult a dietician
Can meditation reduce fatigue?	The right medication or combination of medications can make you more functional	Consult your physician
Have you evaluated your daily routines at home and work?	Energy conservation strategies can help you do things more efficiently	Consult an occupational therapist
Are you using the assistive devices you need?	Many devices can reduce the energy required for daily activities	Consult an occupational therapist
What are your cognitive strengths (and weaknesses)?	You can learn to build on your strengths and compensate for your weaknesses	Consult a neuropsychologist
Do you have a plan for organizing your daily activities?	Developing appropriate routines can increase your productivity	Consult an occupational therapist or speech-language pathologist
Do you ask for help when you need it?	Delegating tasks will give you more time and energy	See chapter 12

Do-It-Yourself Help

As with many people with MS, you may prefer to develop your own plans. Resources are certainly available for those who wish to do this. The National Multiple Sclerosis Society maintains an excellent Web site with educational material, research updates, and information about local resources. Another source of information is the popular press. In today's society, you are not alone in needing to manage your time and energy. There are a number of excellent resources written for the general public.

For example, Loehr and Schwartz (2003) suggest that the key to "full engagement" is to manage energy by balancing stress with periods of recovery. In another bestseller, David Allen (2001) suggests that your ability to get things done is directly proportional to your ability to relax. Further, he recommends that your stress can be reduced if you develop a "collection" system for the various things that you are going to do. Using a dependable system of reminders clears your mind, allows you to focus on accomplishing things, and ultimately reduces stress.

Caregivers

It may be necessary at some point for you to obtain ongoing assistance from a caregiver to get things done. Caregivers can be family members, friends, relatives, paid help, or a combination of all of these. Taking this step doesn't necessarily mean that you will have a loss of independence. For successful and productive interactions with your caregiver(s), you may want to consider the following suggestions. (See chapter 12 for more details.)

Write a job description so that roles and responsibilities will be clear. Writing things down also will give both you and the caregiver a reference point. It is important to set guidelines about your important concerns (e.g., privacy or finance issues), and maintain as much as possible of your personal style.

Professional Help

Finally, consultation with professionals can be an excellent place to start seeking caregiving help. A review of table 2.2 will provide you with a series of suggestions. For example, consulting a physician who specializes in MS is a good way to learn about medications to enhance energy. Again, table 2.2 only provides examples; your local or the National Multiple Sclerosis Society can provide you with an appropriate referral based upon your clearly stated needs.

Conclusion

Getting things done is the work of living. In this chapter, we've outlined some of the aspects of MS that may challenge your ability to work—to get things done. Despite these challenges, it's clear from the many people with MS whom we've interviewed that taking charge of your time and energy allows you to continue to do the things that you value. It is critical for you to set your own priorities, become aware of possible triggers for physical problems, and construct and evaluate a set of strategies that works for you.

CHAPTER 3

Perspectives on Psychotherapy

Dawn M. Ehde, Ph.D.

WHAT IS PSYCHOTHERAPY?

Taking an active role in your own care is part of living fully. This is not only for your physical well-being but also for your emotional health. For example, by reading this book and doing the exercises in it, you are taking an active role in your care. You are trying to learn how to better manage the challenges that your multiple sclerosis (MS) presents.

Sometimes, however, people with MS find it helpful to seek professional help for aid in coping with the many challenges that MS brings.

Professional psychotherapy can be defined in this way: It is a relationship in which one person obtains professional assistance from another for the purpose of bringing about some change in the feelings, thoughts, attitudes, and behavior of the person seeking help. Sometimes, a person will go into therapy knowing changes are needed but doesn't know how to go about making them. The therapist's job is to help that person figure this out, develop options, and aid in making a plan for change.

Types of Therapists

If you live in an urban area, you will have a number of options when seeking a therapist. In rural areas, however, there are fewer practicing professionals. If you live in a rural area, you may want to commute to see a therapist who has a specific type of training or therapeutic orientation. If this entails considerable traveling, you may want to consider an initial meeting or two and then opt for counseling over the telephone. In the last two decades this type of counseling has become increasingly popular.

Examples of individuals trained to provide different kinds of psychotherapy follow below:

Psychologists

A psychologist has a doctoral degree, typically, a Ph.D. or Psy.D., in psychology from an accredited university. This may mean the person has studied at a university for seven or eight years, or even more. In many states, to legally call oneself a "psychologist," one must have a license to practice psychology, which involves passing an examination, a review of credentials, and, often, oral examinations and interviews. Rehabilitation psychologists specialize in an area of psychology that also has trained them in the implications of having a disability such as MS. These psychologists tend to be members of Division 22, Rehabilitation Psychology, the American Psychological Association.

Registered or Certified Counselor, Marriage, Family, and Child (MFC) Counselors

Typically, these counselors have earned either a master's or, in some states, a bachelor's degree in a counseling field or psychology. Because state laws covering counselors vary considerably from state to state, there is no standard description of the kind of training, examination, or credential review (if any) required by the state in order to practice. Professionals may be registered or certified as counselors or as a marriage, family, and child (MFC) counselor with a family systems orientation. Check your state's licensing department regarding counselors if you have any questions.

Clinical Social Workers

Clinical social workers have a master's degree in social work (MSW) and a state license as a clinical social worker. Some of these individuals work at hospitals or outpatient clinics and have a part-time practice in psychotherapy while others are employed with full-time practices.

Psychiatrists

Psychiatrists are medical doctors who after finishing medical school did a four-year psychiatric residency in a hospital. They may or may not have a psychotherapy emphasis in their work but they can prescribe medications for anxiety, depression, and other mood disorders which can be helpful, often as a complement to therapy.

Pastoral Counselors

Some members of the clergy like ministers, priests, rabbis, and so forth have had training as pastoral counselors. They may have a strong religious orientation but some of them make very good therapists indeed. Frequently, they don't charge for their services or they may have a sliding-scale fee in a private practice, depending on the client's ability to pay.

TYPES OF THERAPY

There are many different types and styles of therapy. Which type you use will depend on your preferences and the training and orientation of your therapist. *Orientation* refers to the underlying theory that the therapist subscribes to, which affects the therapist's style, focus, and techniques.

Some of the most common types of therapy are described below. This listing is obviously not meant to be comprehensive; it is intended to give you an overview of the major schools of thought among practitioners of psychotherapy today.

Cognitive Behavioral Therapy

Cognitive behavioral therapy (CBT) emphasizes learning and how "faulty learning" can cause problems in your life. It focuses on your current situation as more important than your past, and its main purpose is to demonstrate to you how your habitual thinking patterns affect your present emotions and behavior.

The theoretical basis of CBT is that many problems stem from irrational and dysfunctional thoughts, ideas, and beliefs, and that these all strongly affect feelings and behaviors. The goal is to modify your dysfunctional thinking so that positive changes in your emotions and behaviors can take place. CBT often involves homework and practicing new behaviors as integral parts of the therapy. The emphasis is on improving your coping skills and abilities.

Psychodynamic/Psychoanalytic Therapy (Insight-Oriented Therapy)

This therapeutic approach is based on the idea that much dysfunctional behavior stems from unconscious impulses and conflicts that developed and were repressed during early childhood. This form of therapy helps clients to bring repressed feelings into conscious awareness. The goal is to work with these new insights over time, with the final goal to modify behavior. Dream interpretation is often a component in this therapy. Due to the emphasis on unconscious impulses and conflicts, the therapy may be intensive, and require more than one therapy session a week.

Humanistic Existential Therapy

The emphasis in humanistic existential therapy is placed on the client's built-in abilities to achieve self-fulfillment. There is a focus on self-awareness and self-acceptance, but the emphasis is more on the present than the past, and on the options and decisions we all must make in our lives.

THERAPY FORMATS

There are a number of different formats in which therapy can be provided. The format you choose can relate to both your therapy needs and your ability to pay for it. Individual psychotherapy sessions are the most common, but based on the problems you have been encountering, other formats may be as helpful as individual sessions. As a person with MS, you may start therapy on your own to deal with issues relating to anxiety, depression, loss of self-esteem, anger, and so forth. It then may be helpful to bring your significant oth... ...to deal with emerging issues, such as the challenges your car... ...ions, or the issues related to your changing abilities to love and ...

...rt, and the high cost of therapy, you may find that group the... ...lp groups (ideally led by a skilled facilitator—who is often a p...

...ek Therapy?

You may seek therapy for a number of reasons. It is a well-known fact that emotional and physical health are interconnected and frequently interdependent. Please check (✓) any of the reasons listed below for seeking therapy that apply to you.

You may consider therapy if you:

____ Feel hopeless or worthless most of the time.

____ Feel overwhelmed by your situation and are unsure of what to do about it.

____ Your emotions, such as stress, sadness, anxiety, or anger, make it hard for you to do what you want to do from day to day.

____ You are doing things that may harm your health, such as neglecting to take your medications, drinking too much alcohol, abusing drugs, or staying in bed all the time.

____ Your emotions or actions are harming your relationships with others.

____ You can't make any progress at work, school, or in other important areas of your life.

____ Individuals you trust, such as a physician or family member, have advised you to seek help.

____ You want to learn more about yourself and how to grow as a person who also happens to have MS.

____ Other

Checking only one reason above can be a valid reason for seeking psychotherapy, but if you've checked several, your need to begin a course of therapy should be apparent to you.

Living with a chronic disease like MS can be life-changing. For some, their identities as people can start to be all about the disease. If you see your primary identity as someone with MS, you may wish to consider therapy to help you learn how to live as someone who happens to have MS.

HOW TO FIND A THERAPIST

Depending on where you live, your preferences, and your resources, finding a therapist can be a challenging process. It is a highly personal decision, too, because a therapist who works well with a friend of yours may not be a good choice for you. For people with MS, however, there are several resources that can help to focus your search. Before you start looking we recommend that you first consider the following issues.

What to Consider Before You Start Looking for a Psychotherapist

The following list is not meant to be exhaustive, but it should give you a framework for choosing a psychotherapist who can work well with your issues.

WORKSHEET 6:   CONSIDERATIONS FOR CHOOSING A PSYCHOTHERAPIST

What type of counseling approach would I like my therapist to use? _____

_____

Do I want my therapist to have a certain educational or training background? _____

_____

Is it important to me that my therapist has experience with MS or at least with physical disabilities? ____

_____

Are there things about the therapist's office or location that are important to me? _____

_____

How can I pay for this therapy? Will my health insurance or HMO plan cover it? _____

_____

Where to Look

Armed with the information that you've clarified on worksheet 6, you now need to find your psychotherapist. The resource points below will help you in your search.

Your healthcare provider. Ask your primary care physician and other health care providers for referrals to therapists who are familiar with MS. If you are seen by an MS specialist such as a *neurologist* (a physician who specializes in the nervous system) or a *physiatrist* (a physician who specializes in physical medicine), he or she is likely to know a therapist who can treat you. Be sure to ask your physician what he or she knows about the therapists they recommend and why they recommend them!

MS community resources. In most large urban areas, there are several community resources that can help you find a therapist. For example, the National Multiple Sclerosis Society can suggest mental health professionals who understand MS. To access this help, contact your local chapter or call 800-FIGHT-MS (800-344-4867). The Multiple Sclerosis Association of America also has a toll-free help line (800-532-7667) that may offer you ideas or strategies for finding a therapist familiar with MS. Both of these organizations can also help you find support groups, telephone networks, and so forth in your area.

Other people with MS. When you have MS, one of the best ways to find a therapist is to ask others with MS. If, currently, you don't know any others with MS, attend a support group or an informational workshop on MS, where you are likely to meet others with MS who have also sought therapy. (Call your local hospital for suggestions about informational workshops.) If you find someone who highly recommends a particular therapist, ask him or her the reasons for the recommendation.

Your friends and family. Ask close friends and family members for their recommendations. You may be surprised to find out how many people you know who have been in therapy. Again, if you find someone who highly recommends a particular therapist, ask him or her the reasons.

Local, county, or state mental health departments/agencies. Although they do not specialize in treating persons with MS, your local or state mental health agencies are another potentially excellent resource for finding a therapist. Look in your local phone book for the names of community mental health agencies. Call them for recommendations for a psychotherapist, or to find out if you are eligible for therapy at their organization, or for the names of organizations that do provide such services. If you have a low income and don't have health insurance coverage for therapy, a community mental health center may be an important option for you to explore; they often provide services based on financial need.

Professional organizations. Many professional organizations have referral services that provide information and names of licensed mental health providers. Some of these providers may offer "pro bono" (free) or sliding-scale fees. For example, to find a licensed psychologist, you can contact the American Psychological Association at 800-964-2000, and then a 411 information-operator will use your zipcode to locate and connect you with your area's referral resource.

If you have cognitive problems (e.g., issues with thinking quickly, memory concerns, and so forth) tell the referral resource about your concerns. In some cases, neuropsychologists who conduct therapy may be good choices because they can better understand your issues in the therapy session, can help to clarify these concerns (see chapter 10), and might be able to help you with useful recommendations.

Your church, synagogue, or religious institution. Ask at your church or synagogue whether they provide therapy services, specifically, whether the cleric is trained in psychotherapy or as a pastoral counselor. Some religious institutions have part-time psychotherapists and provide free or sliding-scale fee schedules. Some religious groups support psychotherapy treatment groups that serve specific areas.

Universities. You may be able to obtain low-cost therapy from a university or school that trains therapists. Some university psychology, counseling, or social work departments have counseling centers where graduate students-in-training provide therapy to those in need of it at no or low cost while supervised by faculty members. If you choose this option, be sure to ask about the training experience of the therapist as well as the amount and type of supervision he or she receives from an experienced provider/faculty member and that person's background.

Questions to ask. Hopefully, after investigating your options, you will wind up with the names of several therapists. When you have a list of options, ask the prospective therapist for the opportunity, either by phone or in person, to ask several questions. Interviewing your potential therapists will help you to make an informed decision about who may best work collaboratively with you. A list of questions to ask a potential therapist appears in the worksheet below.

WORKSHEET 7:   CONSIDERATIONS FOR INTERVIEWING A THERAPIST

Questions to Ask Prospective Therapists

Availability

What is your current availability for taking on new clients? _____

_____

Financial

What are your fees? _____

Do you accept my insurance? (Be prepared to inform the therapist about your specific plan.) _____

How does your billing procedure work? _____

_____

Do you have a sliding-scale fee? (If this is important to you.) _____

What is your policy on charging for cancellations or missed appointments? _____

_____

Education and Licensure

What degree do you have? _____

From where is your degree? _____

How long have you been practicing? _____

Are you licensed? _____

Logistical

Is your office wheelchair accessible? (If needed.) _____

Do you use air-conditioning in the summer? (If relevant to heat tolerance.) _____

How close to your office is parking? _____

How long are typical appointments? _____

Could we teleconference some sessions? (If appropriate, e.g., distance.) _____

Experience

What is your expertise? _____

What is your theoretical orientation? _____

How many people who have MS have you seen? _____

How well did you work with people who have MS? _____

_____

Can you give me some examples of clients you've had (no names) with hidden or neurological disabilities? (Ask this only if the therapist has not treated a client with MS.) _____

_____

Knowledge About and Attitudes Toward Those with MS

What is your understanding of MS? _____

What is your understanding of how MS affects a person's emotions? _____

_____

What do you think are the unique challenges for people with MS? _____

_____

Have you ever personally had a friend or acquaintance with MS? _____

_____

How well did you know that person? _____

Here are my specific questions: (Add your own questions here.)

If a prospective therapist refuses to answer any of your questions, either by phone or during your first appointment, seriously consider looking for someone else. You will do best with a therapist with whom you feel comfortable and with whom you have an honest, trusting, collaborative relationship. It is, however, important to be respectful of the therapist's time and to be polite as you go through your list of questions. A good psychotherapist can be quite busy.

MAKING YOUR CHOICE

Once you've interviewed several prospective therapists and examined your options in terms of finances and convenience, it is time to make your choice. Your choice may be clear; you may have decided that you want to work with one person whom you've interviewed. If you haven't made your choice yet, list the key factors for your choice of psychotherapists from the answers you've generated for worksheet 7:

1.

2.

3.

4.

Based on the above, my top therapist choice(s) are:

_____ , _____ , _____ .

Now you need to assess the therapist's availability, and make that appointment.

WHAT TO EXPECT FROM THERAPY

In the initial interview (or consultation), the therapist should disclose to you the relevant information about his or her training, background, experience, and approach to services. Fees and payment arrangements should be clearly stated. Much of this information is usually available on the disclosure sheet you are commonly given at the first appointment. Often, the first session is a consultation. The initial emphases are for the therapist to talk with you to figure out your difficulties, strengths, and goals, and to discuss how you might work together to meet your goals. The first session is a time to decide whether you will feel comfortable with this therapist. Will this therapist and therapeutic approach be helpful to you? The therapist must decide, too, whether he or she can work with you. If not, you should be told why and help should be provided in finding a therapist who may work better with you.

Early sessions are often spent talking about what led you to seek therapy. Sometimes referred to as an "assessment," the therapist will ask you specific questions about your concerns. You may be asked personal questions about your life experiences and family background/experiences.

Sometimes assessment may include having you complete questionnaires or tests. Ask questions if you have any about the purpose of testing. You can also ask for the results to be reviewed with you. (Take notes or tape-record if that seems helpful.) After assessment, set goals; therapy should then focus on helping you gain insight into your problems and how to make changes. The goals of therapy and the definition of a successful outcome should be clear to you.

Sometimes, therapy may involve the therapist listening to you and helping you to clarify your emotions. Other times, it may involve practicing techniques both inside and outside of therapy. For example, relaxation methods and reading assignments can all take place outside of the therapy sessions. Therapists vary on how directive they are. Some will be very directive, others will let you take the lead. Make sure you feel reasonably comfortable with the approach that is used.

Typically, therapy lasts forty-five to sixty minutes a session and may occur on a weekly basis or on a more or less frequent basis. As you progress, you may decide to see your therapist less frequently. It is a good idea to ask your therapist about the length and frequency of therapy that you might expect based on your assessment data and goals. Successful therapy is a collaboration, a two-way process that works best when patients and therapists have an open, collaborative relationship.

After you meet your goals, you may decide further therapy is no longer needed. Some therapists will ask you to return in a few weeks or months for a check-up visit to see how you are doing and to make sure you are maintaining your gains. It is up to you to decide to set this appointment, but it is often a good idea.

You may experience a wide range of emotions when in therapy. You may feel nervous or have difficulty in discussing difficult things. Some days it may be uncomfortable or even "intimidating" to attend your scheduled session because of the emotional material with which you are dealing. Such emotions are normal and can, in fact, be a positive step in your progression. It is best to discuss these concerns with your therapist and to "stay the course."

In sum, the therapeutic relationship must be based on a balance of trust, mutual respect, and openness in dialogue. It can be very helpful to feel empathy from your therapist and to work with one who will respond to your needs/questions within the context of his or her acknowledged limitations. After several weeks of sessions, if you haven't started to experience any benefit, it may be helpful to seek a new therapist after discussing your perceived need for change with the one whom you've been seeing.

WHAT SHOULD NOT HAPPEN IN THERAPY

Your relationship with your therapist should be based on mutual trust and respect. Licensed therapists are expected to adhere to a code of ethics and to the state laws pertaining to the practice of their profession. Some things that should not happen include the following:

- Violation of your privacy/confidentiality (including your records/test data)

- Infringement on your legal or civil rights

- Sexual harassment, inappropriate touching, and/or other relations

- Physical or verbal abuse

- Any form of exploitation

If you think your therapist is acting unethically, you should speak to him or her about your concerns, if you feel safe in doing so. If your therapist does not answer your concerns, you should consider changing to another. You can report the therapist's behavior to the relevant local health professionals' association or state licensing department.

WORKING WITH YOUR THERAPIST: KEY POINTS

Set goals. Be clear with your therapist and yourself about your expectations. Try not to let each other stray from your established objectives. Obviously, this will happen on occasion, but it should not become a common practice.

Be an active, not a passive, participant. Be prepared, rested, and punctual for sessions. Do your homework assignments. The more you put into therapy, the more you will get from it. Before your sessions, give some thought ahead of time to what you want to discuss. If you get to your appointment a few minutes early, you will have time to do this.

Collaborate/Educate on MS. Share with your therapist new information and relevant books on MS. Reference the National Multiple Sclerosis Society's Web site (www.nationalmssociety.org) and discuss the physical, sensory, and cognitive issues that can affect your emotions. This is critical because many good psychotherapists may lack current information on the impact MS can have on an individual's life, and specifically how it is affecting you.

Keep your appointments. Missing therapy appointments is not helpful, as you will best progress if you attend all scheduled sessions. You may also want to move up an appointment if you are leaving town or otherwise discuss how you might make up missed sessions with your therapist.

Dreading your appointments. If you notice yourself dreading attending therapy sessions, or missing appointments regularly, think about what your reasons may be. It could be more than simple situational inconveniences, illness, and so forth. It may be a sign that you are avoiding dealing with issues or that, for some reason, you are frustrated with your therapist. These issues need to be brought up and discussed. It is important to remember that some of this short-term emotional pain is part of the process to a long-term adjustment to MS that you must undergo.

Review your progress. Share your concerns with your therapist as they come up. You may need to adjust your goals. After a few sessions, you should feel that the therapeutic experience is collaborative and that you feel comfortable with your therapist. A certain amount of time should be spent reviewing your progress with the therapist.

If you find yourself thinking about stopping therapy, discuss the matter with your therapist first. If you think you have met your goals, tell the therapist. If you feel stuck, discuss that with the therapist.

DOES THERAPY WORK?

Yes. It does! Most of what we know about the effectiveness of therapy comes from studies done on those with only emotional concerns or on those with other health problems, such as cancer. This research suggests that therapy can be effective in helping individuals with chronic illnesses feel better in many ways. It can reduce depression, anxiety, and stress. Therapy has also been shown to improve health (Ehde and Bombardier 2005).

The few studies looking at the effectiveness of therapy among persons with MS suggest that therapy is also beneficial to persons with MS (Ehde and Bombardier 2005). We also believe that it can help MS-related symptoms such as pain and fatigue.

Conclusion

We hope that this chapter has provided you with a comfortable framework for finding a therapist if you feel the need. Therapy support can be very helpful, not only in dealing with crisis, but in charting new directions and in making your adjustment to living with MS. There are a number of options and fee structures (including sliding scale and pro bono work). Try not to sit on the sidelines in emotional pain. Take advantage of some of the great resources that are out there. Our very best wishes to you in this process.

CHAPTER 4

Health-Promoting Behaviors

Charles H. Bombardier, Ph.D.

TAKING CONTROL OF YOUR HEALTH

In this time of rapid advances in technology and medicine it may be tempting to see your health as the responsibility of doctors and other medical specialists. It's easy to lose sight of the simple yet powerful things you can do to enhance your own health. In this chapter you will find a number of options about reclaiming control over your own health, in spite of having multiple sclerosis (MS). You will learn how to identify when you are ready to change key health behaviors and the areas where you are most ready to change. You will also learn how to tailor your health-promotion efforts to fit your specific stage in the change process.

We will explore how to work through several very common ways that people get stuck when they are trying to make changes. Some of these "stuck" places may be well-known to you by phrases like the following:

- People say you are "in denial." What to do when you don't want to change.

- You feel trapped in ambivalence. "I want to change, but..."

- You were doing fine, but you've "relapsed." Two steps forward, one step back. By working with, rather than against, your stage of change, you can move ahead.

Finally, we will look at several specific areas of health promotion in detail and provide you with suggestions to consider and activities to engage in for each area.

HEALTH PROMOTION: WHAT IT IS AND ISN'T

Doing what you can to improve your own health is called *health promotion*. Health-promoting activities come in two flavors: actions you can take to stop doing certain behaviors that will improve your health; and actions you can take to start doing certain behaviors to improve your health. Some health-promoting activities are just common sense. But, of course, we all know that we don't always do what we know we should. Other health-promoting activities may seem counterintuitive. Moreover, there are areas where we've only recently learned something about what seems to work.

Good examples of behaviors to stop doing are the common addictions: overeating, smoking tobacco, abusing alcohol, and misusing prescription or over-the-counter medications. We will discuss each of these common unhealthy habits below.

There are many things you can start doing to improve your health. For example, you could (1) start taking *course-altering medications,* such as an immunomodulator for your MS or a medication for managing spasticity, either for the first time or to renew your commitment to fully adhere to the dosage schedule for a course-altering medication that you may have started and stopped. (2) You can start exercising more often or adopt a more active lifestyle. (3) You can get serious about managing your fatigue. (4) You can learn more effective ways to cope with stress and anxiety. And (5) you can learn to ask for help and begin utilizing your social support network. Some actions you can do on your own. Some you can do with a friend or family member. Other actions require your doctor, rehabilitation therapist, or other healthcare provider to be your partner.

HEALTH-PROMOTING ACTIVITIES WORK WELL FOR PEOPLE WITH MS

Dr. Alexa Stuifbergen, a nursing researcher in Austin, Texas, has studied health-promotion activities in people with MS for years. In a 1997 study, she measured the extent to which women with MS engaged in various health-promoting activities including keeping physically active, eating nutritious diets, taking responsibility for their health, improving their interpersonal relations, focusing on meaning or spiritual growth, and managing their stress. She also measured each woman's physical abilities and quality of life (Stuifbergen and Roberts 1997).

The results of her research are shown in figure 4.1. She found that two factors heavily influence the quality of life for women with MS: that is, their physical abilities and their heath-promoting activities. Notice that the arrow between physical abilities and health-promoting activities is very thin. That means that people with milder MS, as well as those with more severe MS, all benefit equally from health-promoting activities.

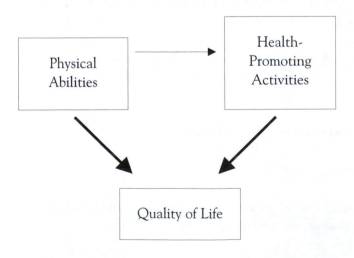

Figure 4.1: Health promotion and MS.

Question: Which health-promoting activity do you think gives the most "bang for the buck?" Answer: Exercise. Think about it. Aerobic exercise in people with MS has been shown to improve strength, decrease fatigue, improve mood, decrease anger, and improve social interactions, home management, and recreational activities. Exercise packs a powerful punch. Keep this in mind later when you think about your options for improving your health.

THE STAGES OF CHANGE

Until recently, we've tended to view people as either ready to change or not ready, like a light switch that is either On or Off. In many cases, those not ready to change were labeled as "resistant" or "in denial" when they did not change in the ways that others thought they should. In the past two decades, we've come to a deeper understanding of change processes and, hopefully, a more useful and compassionate view of it.

For example, James Prochaska and his colleagues (1994) became tired of armchair theories about how people change. They decided instead to study how average people create change naturally. They studied people who were trying to quit smoking, lose weight, and start exercising. They even studied those who make New Year's resolutions to try to gain insight into natural change processes.

One of their discoveries was that change is often a more complex process than it was initially thought to be. They found there are several common stages that people who want to change go through, and that, on their way to making and sustaining behavioral change, they tended to go through a progression of these stages. What follows are brief descriptions of the stages of change that Prochaska and his colleagues identified in their study.

Stage 1: Precontemplation

Precontemplation refers to the stage when you are not changing, not interested in change, and perhaps even defensive about not changing, especially if confronted about your need to change. In precontemplation, you may be unaware or underaware of the need to change in a particular way. You might be in precontemplation out of a sense of hopelessness, or of not wanting to feel controlled, or from ignorance, or just out of reluctance. Other people may be concerned or worried about you, but you can't see a need to change. You even may avoid reading or talking about the topic.

Stage 2: Contemplation

Contemplation is the stage in which people are ambivalent about change. That is, the pros and cons of changing seem about evenly balanced, leaving the person stuck. In the contemplation stage, people often think that they should change in some area, but they don't get to the point of actually changing what they do.

Ambivalence about change is extremely common and can last for many years. If you repeatedly think about changing in a particular area but never get around to it, or you rationalize your way out of it, or you decide that changing is just not worth the trouble it will take, you are probably in the contemplation stage.

Stage 3: Preparation

In the preparation stage, you have decided to change, you've made plans to change, but have not yet actually initiated the change. For example, smokers who are determined to stop may set a quit date, dieters who are determined to change their eating habits may stock up on different and healthier foods, and people determined to become more fit may figure out how they are going to fit new forms of exercise into their daily or weekly schedules.

You are in the preparation stage if you plan to begin a new health-promoting activity within the next thirty days.

Stage 4: Action

The action stage is when behavioral change really begins. Everything up until this point has been mental changes. Now the person starts to do something new, or perhaps stops doing something old (which still involves doing something new). The action stage corresponds to using new behaviors that started up and have been sustained for up to six months, that is, long enough for the new behavior to become a relatively well-established habit.

Have there been any new health-promotion activities you've begun and sustained within the past six months?

Stage 5: Relapse

Relapse obviously refers to a return to previous behavior patterns that were in place before actions were taken to try to change. Recently, relapse has become recognized as an almost universal stage of change rather than as an anomaly or a failure to change. Most people initiate behavior change and then relapse several times before the change is maintained successfully. For example, most smokers quit four to eight times before maintaining their status as nonsmokers (Prochaska, Norcross, and DiClemente 1992).

Think about any new healthy habits you tried to acquire in the past six months. Try to recall any relapses that occurred, such as not sticking to a diet or picking up smoking again, or giving up on a walking program.

Stage 6: Maintenance

After a new action has been successfully followed for about six months, the person is said to enter the maintenance stage. In this stage, a habit has been formed, but maintaining it over the long haul is less certain.

YOUR STAGE OF CHANGE PROFILE

Worksheets 8 and 9 below list a large number of potential health-promoting activities you can consider. Worksheet 8 lists actions you can start doing. Worksheet 9 lists actions you could stop doing. For each item on both worksheets, ask yourself, "What stage of change am I in?" Check the stage of change column that corresponds with your stage of change for each health-promoting activity.

If, for example, you are a nonsmoker, put your check in the maintenance column. There is a space in each category for you to fill in another idea. Write in any other health-promoting activities that you are contemplating, preparing for, doing, maintaining, or that have relapsed.

Be Kind to Yourself

While you fill in the worksheets, try to appreciate the progress you may have already made. Maybe you'll recognize an item where you were previously in denial, and now you are contemplating some sort of positive change. Perhaps you had long-standing ambivalence about initiating a change, and now you've finally reached the point of taking action.

It is especially important to appreciate areas where you changed and then relapsed, because even though you relapsed, you did make a positive change for a certain period of time. Furthermore, there are usually lessons to learn from a relapse that will help you the next time.

It's also a good idea to think about whether your change efforts are focused on just a few areas or spread out over many areas. Which changes are you most excited about? Which ones are looming? Which ones do you dread?

WORKSHEET 8: A MENU OF HEALTH-PROMOTING OPTIONS

Health-Promoting Strategy: Behaviors to begin or improve. Specify as best you can.	Precontemplation	Contemplation	Preparation	Action	Relapse	Maintenance
Energy conservation						
Cut down on less important activities						
Work smarter (organize, prioritize, create efficiencies, start earlier, etc.)						
Ask for help/delegate						
Pace yourself; break down large activities into smaller ones						
Other						
Energy recharging						
Make time for rest, relaxation, naps						
Improve sleep quality or amount						

Have fun; maintain or seek new hobbies and recreation						
Other						
Energy enhancement						
Exercise (strength, endurance, stretching)						
Increase physical activity, e.g., walking, water aerobics, etc.						
Other						
Maximize medical management						
Fatigue-reducing medications						
Disease-modifying medications						
Antispasticity medications						
Improve adherence to current medications						
Antidepressant medications						
Bladder function medications						
Learn more about disease or treatments						
Discuss problems with healthcare provider or consultant						
Other						
Manage psychological challenges						
Use stress/worry management techniques						
Rediscover meaning and purpose in life through psychological or spiritual counseling						
Challenge hopeless or negativistic thinking						
Reaffirm core values or spirituality						
Replace passive with active coping skills						
Other						

WORKSHEET 9: REDUCING NEGATIVE BEHAVIORS						
Health-Promoting Strategy: Behaviors to stop doing or cut down.	Precontemplation	Contemplation	Preparation	Action	Relapse	Maintenance
Smoking						
Alcohol use						
Illicit drug use						
Medication misuse						
Excessive independence						
Overactivity						
Excessive exposure to heat, humidity, or cold						
Unhealthy eating habits						
Poor sleeping habits						
Other						

WHERE AND HOW TO START THE CHANGE PROCESS?

You can really start anywhere and, as you will see, you are thinking about, making or preparing for, or relapsing from change all the time in several areas. One good place to start would be an area about which you are most enthused right now and where you can see the most payoff for your work. On the other hand, if there is no particular area for which you feel any enthusiasm, you can start in any area.

You can make significant progress even when you are in the precontemplation stage about changing in an important area, perhaps an area where others have implied you "should" change. Or maybe there is an area in which you feel resigned, reluctant, or even resistant to change. Yet, way in the back of your mind, you may also have the suspicion that your life could be improved in this area.

Keeping a Journal

It would be a good idea to start keeping a separate journal while you read and work with this book. Of course, there are many worksheets within the text for you to write down your thoughts about specific subjects; however, there are also many instances where the text encourages you to think about something specific. As a general rule, when you write your thoughts down, the writing clarifies the material about which you are thinking. Also, a separate journal will allow you to expand and elaborate on anything of importance that comes up for you while you are working with this book.

THE PRECONTEMPLATION STAGE

One place to start thinking and writing about might be to simply notice any psychological defenses you use to maintain your state of not changing. Precontemplators tend to deny or minimize the negative consequences of their unhealthy behaviors. Others rationalize or make repeated excuses for not changing in a particular area. Some blame their inability to change on others or on external circumstances over which they believe they have no control.

Noticing your defenses can lead to a healthier attitude about your responsibility for not changing. There is something more honest and empowering about changing your belief from "I can't do that," or "If only I could do that," to "Right now, I am choosing not to do that." The fact is, it's your life and you don't have to change in any way that you don't wish to change. Only you can decide if changing is worth the risk and effort. No one can force you to change.

Simply to understand yourself better, you could also take out your journal and try listing the benefits you get from not changing. You might be avoiding working too hard, exposing yourself to criticism, or risking failure. Or you might have an entirely different set of reasons for not wanting to change. But it would be a good idea to know what they are.

Another way to start the change process might be to think about the area where you don't want to change and project yourself five to ten years into the future. Ask yourself, "Where will I be ten years down the road if I continue not changing in this area and how does that fit with what I want to be or become as a person?" This question can help you see whether the benefits of not changing now may shift over time. Ultimately, it's best not to get stuck in a battle with yourself over not changing in some particular area. We hope that you identified an area (or areas) where changing holds more interest for you. So let's move on to the next stages of change.

THE CONTEMPLATION AND PREPARATION STAGES

Moving into the preparation stage after contemplation involves understanding and changing the balance between the pros and cons associated with the specific behavior. Doing the decisional balance exercise below in worksheet 10 provides a good way for contemplators to begin moving into the preparation stage. The decisional balance expands your old pros and cons for changing to include the benefits of not changing and the costs of changing versus the benefits of changing.

Moreover, to completely understand all the factors, these pros and cons of changing can be analyzed in terms of short-term versus long-term costs and benefits. You can use worksheet 10 to examine an area where you may be stuck in the contemplation stage. Discovering more potential positive benefits of changing can be the surest way to move yourself toward action. If you can identify five, ten, or even more potential benefits you may receive from changing, either short- or long-term, the greater your chances are of moving toward action.

WORKSHEET 10: THE DECISIONAL BALANCE

Write the change being contemplated here: _____

_____

After you've written in the change you are considering making, fill in the specific pros and cons that would result from making that change. Fill in the short-term costs of changing and the short-term benefits of not changing. Then fill in the short-term costs of not changing and the short-term benefits of changing. After you've completed filling in that part of the worksheet, go through the same analysis for the long-term costs and benefits of changing and not changing.

Cons of Change		Pros of Change	
Short-term costs of change	Short-term benefits of *not* changing	Short-term costs of *not* changing	Short-term benefits of change
1.	1.	1.	1.
2.	2.	2.	2.
3.	3.	3.	3.
Long-term costs of change	Long-term benefits of *not* changing	Long-term costs of *not* changing	Long-term benefits of change
1.	1.	1.	1.
2.	2.	2.	2.
3.	3.	3.	3.

In this preparation stage, you can put more teeth in your plans in several ways. You can shore up your motivation to change by writing down your most important reasons for changing, especially the benefits. Be specific about what you will do, and tell others about your plans. Set a start date and make a list of the things you need to get ready to begin the change you are preparing for.

THE ACTION STAGE

Once you are in the action stage, actually making the changes, reward yourself. Tell others about what you've accomplished; chart your progress. Don't forget that many people relapse back into their old behaviors. Make a crisis plan for what you will do if you should experience a relapse. That way you can keep a brief lapse from turning into a more extended relapse.

Crisis Plans for Relapses

As a rule, a crisis plan involves contacting a trusted friend who supports and accepts you unconditionally when you are in the action stage. Explain to your friend that you are making an important change in your life but you may have a relapse, and you want to enlist your friend's future help if the need arises. Tell your friend that, if you do relapse, you won't need criticism or lectures to worsen your guilt.

Together, you and your friend can normalize your relapse, review the main reasons you wanted to change, appreciate the changes you did make, and see where you want to go from there. If you have relapsed previously, this would be a good time to look for the specific triggers that led to the relapse, and perhaps to modify your goals or strategy in accordance.

If you are in relapse now, take heart. You are in good company.

Relapse can be a failure with a silver lining if you make the effort to find your triggers. Pay attention to the feelings, situations, people, or events that led to relapse and you can learn a lot about how to prevent it the next time. Sometimes you have to look back several steps, before the relapse took place, to see where the factors leading to relapse began.

Identify Your Relapse Triggers

Identifying your triggering factors allows you to anticipate and plan to cope with those situations in new ways. First, notice how you felt after your relapse. Guilty? Demoralized? Frustrated? These negative emotions and others are common reactions to relapse. To combat this tendency think about and try to appreciate the progress you did make before the relapse occurred. You got to the point of making a change, got started, and made some headway. How did it feel to do that? Reflect on the things you are proud of and about the changes you did make, regardless of how long they lasted. Understand that people rarely make significant changes without relapsing along the way. When you feel guilty or ashamed about a relapse, remind yourself that this is normal, happens to everyone, and is instructive as a test-run toward your goal.

Next, think about the specific situations, events, people, or feelings that preceded your relapse. Which of these factors triggered you to give up your efforts to change? How did you cope with it at the time?

Finally, what are some alternative ways you can handle these relapse triggers in the future? It is best to plan ahead how you would like to handle this situation in the future. Get out your journal and write down what you will do in the event that you need to cope with this or similar situations in the future. You increase your chances of successfully changing if you write down what you will do the next time. If you choose not to write it down, then tell the friend you enlisted for support in the event of a relapse.

THE MAINTENANCE STAGE

After you have made it into the maintenance phase, you have six months of change under your belt. You have truly been successful. Congratulations! A question that now arises is that of your lifestyle balance. If your lifestyle change is based primarily on self-denial or on considerable effort without tangible rewards, the change may not last as long as you desire. Therefore, it is important to balance self-denial and hard work with healthy pleasures and rewards. If your lifestyle change involves stopping or cutting back on some pleasurable activity, you must come up with other newer, healthier ways to reward yourself. Take pleasure breaks, call a friend just to chat, or each time you take that injection or do that exercise, contribute some money, even if it's only a dollar, toward a special purchase you want to make. Substitute healthier habits for less healthy ones; for example, buy some of your favorite ice cream or chocolate instead of cigarettes or alcohol.

HEALTH PROMOTION: FOUR CORE AREAS

Here, we will take a look at four general types of health-promoting activities that are beneficial for people with MS: exercise and activity; managing fatigue; coping better with stress and anxiety; and coping better with alcohol or other drug misuse.

Exercise and Activity

Sara was an avid golfer, a wife, and mother when she was diagnosed with MS. In the early 1990s her doctor's advice regarding how to cope with the fatigue was in keeping with then-current clinical lore, "rest and conserve your energy." Sara gave up golf, limited her other enjoyable but nonessential activities, and saved what energy she had for key family responsibilities. She was plagued by fatigue, the unpredictable good days and bad days, and the fear that overactivity would worsen her fatigue or bring on a full-blown exacerbation. She missed golf, she missed her old life, and she felt trapped by her symptoms and fear of relapse.

In the past ten years, medical research has turned upside down how we think about coping with MS. Now, we know that by resting and avoiding activities, Sara's muscles were weakened and shrank, her fatigue worsened, her mood, self-esteem, and self-confidence all plummeted further down than they might have, had she been given different advice. That is, some symptoms Sara suffered from were caused by inactivity and deconditioning, not by MS.

Fortunately, Sara volunteered for a study that supported her efforts to build back her strength and endurance. She started where she was at; walking for about ten minutes several times a week. By systematically increasing her walking distance over the course of several months she was eventually able to play nine holes of golf and enjoy it. After several months, she was invited to spend a weekend playing golf. She played several eighteen-hole rounds of golf in two days. Sara was exhausted, of course, but she was also very happy. She had reclaimed a part of her life she thought she had lost.

When it comes to exercise, you have many options to choose from. Most people can find something that fits well with their lifestyle. Some people are able to enjoy more vigorous aerobic activities, such as jogging, cycling, swimming, or aerobics. Others may want to focus more on strength-building using weights or machines. Still others prefer or are limited to stretching and range-of-motion activities such as yoga or Pilates.

We tend to think of exercise only as going to the pool or gym, jogging down a pathway, or playing a sport. All of these are great. Yet, every movement can be considered exercise, giving rise to the popularity of *lifestyle exercise*. When you incorporate exercise into your lifestyle, that means walking to the store rather than driving. It means parking a few blocks from your destination and walking the rest of the way. Or climbing stairs rather than taking the elevator. Gardening, mowing the lawn, shopping, even housework are all forms of exercise. The list of lifestyle activities involving movement and exercise could continue for another paragraph.

Exercise Tips

Here are some tips for successful exercisers. Although exercise generally is considered safe for people with MS, talking with your doctor about your plan, before embarking on an exercise program, can provide reassurance and useful advice. Think about what you are already doing and expand on that. Recall activities you used to enjoy and think about ways to reclaim them a bit at a time. Make it fun and your motivation will last. Start from where you are, even if that is at zero, and set small attainable goals. If you can walk only fifty feet before you are fatigued, don't lament; start with that today and set your goal to improve slowly, by 5 to 10 percent each time.

Remember, take baby steps. Avoid the self-defeating cycle of overactivity followed by intense fatigue and underactivity by not overdoing it in the first place. Set a reasonable goal and stick to it. When you meet the goal for the day, stop so you don't overdo.

If you can, join classes or others who are already exercising. The commitment and social support can help you stick to your goals when your motivation wanes. Plan for possible heat sensitivity problems by "pre-cooling" in a cool bath before exercising, obtain a cooling vest, stay in the shade, and exercise during cooler times of day or in air-conditioned facilities. Remember to keep hydrated. Experiment and find out what works for you.

If you have been avoiding activities out of fear of exacerbations or sideeffects, make a crisis plan. You might have a friend join you, or you could carry a cell phone and identify someone to call for help if you start to feel bad while you are away from home. Chart your progress and reward yourself when you meet your goals.

Managing Fatigue

Fatigue is almost universal among people with MS and often it can be the most disabling symptom. Fatigue can be "physical" or "mental" or a combination of both. It can be chronic and constant or episodic, often increasing unexpectedly or with exertion. Fatigue can come directly from MS or it can be related to secondary problems with sleep, depression, or medication side effects, as well as to MS-related breathing problems or difficulty moving.

Since 1998, there have been specific guidelines established to help physicians understand how to help manage MS-related fatigue (Kinkel et al. 1998). More research has been done since then and this is an area where partnership with your physician is especially important. Your doctor can help you determine whether your fatigue potentially will be compounded by any of the factors listed above, and whether medications such as amantadine, pemoline, or modafinil might be useful to you.

In addition to working with your doctor there are a number of other ways you can gain some control over your fatigue. Of course, as noted above, one of the most exciting recent discoveries is that aerobic exercise actually improves fatigue in people with MS. There is no reason to doubt that other forms of exercise that build strength or endurance would not also improve fatigue. The reverse also seems to be true, that is, excessive rest and inactivity can make fatigue worse.

There are also a number of energy conservation strategies that you may find beneficial. Use the checklist below to see how many of these strategies you already use and which ones you might consider trying again or improving.

Checklist 5: Fatigue Management

____ I break large tasks into smaller, manageable parts.

____ I reflect on my core values and give priority to activities most meaningful to me.

____ I prioritize tasks and do the most important ones first.

____ I organize tasks first to reduce unnecessary effort.

____ I pace myself by resting or napping before I become overexhausted.

____ I delegate or ask for help with tasks that are either too difficult or have a lower priority for me.

____ I use strategies to prevent, avoid, or reduce overheating.

____ I avoid becoming sedentary and deconditioned.

____ When needed, I modify tasks so I can do them more easily, e.g., while sitting.

____ I maintain a daily schedule and set realistic goals as much as possible.

____ I accept certain limits and help others who rely on me to understand those limits.

____ I reserve my time and energy for recreation, family, and friends.

Better Coping with Stress and Anxiety

A lot of normal, understandable stress comes along with MS. The unpredictability of the disease, and its unexpected overwhelming fatigue or exacerbations can trigger a sense of helplessness and a passive, avoidant, or giving-up style of coping. Although such a response to the stress of MS is understandable, other responses are possible and undoubtedly healthier.

How you cope begins with how you think about your illness and its related stressors. Consider some aspect of having MS that is stressful to you now. Do you think of this aspect of your illness as a threat or a challenge? If a stressor is perceived as a threat, people are prone to become fearful. We become tense and sweat as our body releases stress hormones. Our heart races. To deal with this discomfort, we tend to avoid and otherwise cope passively with this stressor. However, when we perceive stressors as a challenge, we tend to think in terms of problem solving, engaging the stressor, and taking constructive action.

Research has shown that people with MS who use these kinds of active coping fare better (Pakenham 1999). So, the key question is how to change "threats" into "challenges."

You could start by picking up your journal and writing down a list of the current threatening aspects of your illness, the events or people you are avoiding, the aspects that make you feel anxious or stressed. It may be that you can't predict when you are going to feel well, so now you avoid making plans altogether. Maybe you've thought about starting on one of the ABC disease-modifying drugs, but you can't bear the thought of self-injection or the possible side effects. Maybe the people in your life don't understand your illness, that you need to ask for help, or that you are withdrawing and becoming depressed about your illness and your life.

After you've made such a list, number each stressful aspect on that list from 1 (the hardest to deal with) down to 5 (the easiest to deal with). *Start with the easiest current threat you have to deal with* and spend a few additional minutes writing down what your biggest fears are about this issue. Pay close attention to the thoughts that come to your mind. Let yourself catastrophize. What makes it a threat? Get down on paper your worst-case scenarios about what might happen if you tried to change in this area. You may become even more stressed doing this journal writing and you may notice the close connections between how you think about things and how you feel emotionally and physically.

Then, work with worksheet 11 to rate how stressed you are on a scale of 0 (not at all) to 100 (as stressed as imaginable). Also rate how much you believe in your worst-case scenarios from 0 to 100 percent.

WORKSHEET 11: MY THREAT LIST		
Describe the top five most threatening aspects of your illness (worst-case scenarios), how stressed you are by each, and how much you believe each will come true.	Stress level 0-100	Belief level 0-100
1.		
2.		
3.		
4.		
5.		

The Opposite of Stress Is Relaxation

The next step in this process is to take a break from all this stress and allow yourself to relax. Get into a comfortable position and practice a calming strategy such as deep abdominal breathing. Or imagine you are in a very peaceful, relaxing place you once visited and try to relive all the sights, sounds, smells, tastes, and other sensations of that experience. Once you have taken some time (at least ten minutes) to relax and enjoy the sense of calmness and ease you can give yourself, then you can allow your mind to shift back to the easiest threat you identified above, and ask yourself the questions you will find in worksheet 12.

WORKSHEET 12:   COPING WITH YOUR THREATS

Note which words or phrases you used that were especially emotional or extreme. Also note your use of words like "always," "never," "should," "must," or "can't," and statements where you catastrophize (imagining the most catastrophic outcome possible), or where you feel hopeless, or helpless.

What is the evidence for the idea that this threat is something I should be stressed and frightened about?

_____

What is the evidence against the idea that this threat is something that is so threatening?

_____

What is the evidence for the belief that I can cope with this threat?

_____

What are some potentially good things that could happen if I deal with this threat differently?

_____

What am I thankful about regarding this threat? E.g., How is my current situation better than it could be?

_____

What aspects of this threat, however small, do I have control over and might be able to change?

_____

What strategies have I used to cope actively with stress in the past that I can apply to this threat?

_____

Once you've had some time to reflect on this "threat" in a calmer state of mind, you may discover, not solutions, but small inroads that will address some aspect of the threat/stressor or a place to start. A glimmer of gratitude for what you have been spared, a foothold where you can achieve a degree of control, an opportunity that you can grasp. With each of these changes in your thinking, your reappraisal of the stressor can lead to a sense of possibility and a challenge that you can take up.

If you have been successful at learning to see your stressor as less of a threat and more of a challenge, you may wish to solidify your insight in some way. You can do this easily by writing down your reappraisal on a small index card, to carry with you or to put up next to the bathroom mirror where you will be sure to see it every day.

Jill's Story

Jill was overwhelmed by all the housework she did, especially the vacuuming, which often led to her becoming overly fatigued. By examining her current appraisal of that situation, she noticed she felt she "should" be able to keep up with the housework. It made her feel "trapped," "guilty," and her family "didn't appreciate" how much effort she had to expend on such household chores. After reflecting on this situation with her therapist, she noticed how the word "should" implied a rigid, somewhat moralistic expectation that she put on herself.

She changed her appraisal to what she came to see as a more accurate view: "MS has made housework much more difficult for me." She wrote this reappraisal down on a small index card that she kept in her wallet. Whenever she started to feel trapped or guilty, she pulled the card out of her wallet and read it over several times.

This simple admission of her difficulties led her to consider a number of possible solutions that were more in line with her core values of being a good mother and wife. She realized it was worth it to ask for help with housework from her family or, if no one had the time, to hire someone to come in and vacuum every other week so that she would have the energy to cook and monitor her son's homework more consistently.

Coping with Alcohol or Other Drug Misuse

People with MS are not immune from problems with using or abusing alcohol or other drugs. Smoking, alcohol use, and misuse of prescription or over-the-counter medications are all potential concerns for people with MS. The use of controlled substances is relevant in the context of health promotion because the negative effects that alcohol or other drugs may have on people with MS may be magnified.

For example, alcohol can cause or contribute to problems with depression. Moreover, heavy alcohol use can make antidepressant medications ineffective. Alcohol or other drug use can alter liver function and change how well your body is able to metabolize other medications, as well. This may cause additional side effects such as increased drowsiness, fatigue, loss of coordination, or balance. Medications that can have bad interactions with alcohol and other drugs include painkillers, antispasticity medications, cold medications, anti-inflammatory drugs (e.g., ibuprofen, naproxen), blood-thinning agents, antibiotics, and antihistamines. Alcohol or other drugs may exacerbate subtle cognitive impairment.

Despite the health risks, people who use alcohol or other drugs are not crazy or weird, they are much like everyone else. They have their reasons to use controlled substances that make sense to them. Therefore, alcohol or drug use cannot be dismissed with a simplistic "Don't do it!" From a health-promoting perspective, what can be helpful is to examine the pros and cons of alcohol or other drug use. If you smoke or use alcohol or other drugs, including overuse of prescription medications, consider going through the following brief exercise:

Exercise: Alcohol or Drug Use in Your Life

Use your journal to do this exercise. First, list all the good things about your use of alcohol or other drugs. What are the perceived benefits to you, physically, mentally and socially? There must be some benefits or you wouldn't be using them.

Next, list the not-so-good aspects about your use of alcohol or other drugs. What concerns do you have about your use, either in the near-term or the long-term, if your use continues as it is now?

Next, take some time to consider how your alcohol or other drug use fits in with who you are and who you want to become. This should reflect your values, your situation, and the important goals you have for yourself in life. Perhaps you are married and have children and want to be a good parent. How does alcohol or drug use fit in with that? Maybe you are unemployed and trying to get back on your feet. Or you may be newly diagnosed with MS and wondering what course this illness will take in your life and whether you have any control over it.

When thinking through these issues, it is important to remember several things. No one can force you to change; it really comes down to what you want for your life. Also, no one can change for you. It's up to you to change if you want to. Don't get bogged down by not wanting to make a particular kind of change you think you should make; for example, deciding to abstain for life. That is a huge decision and only one of the many options open to you. It also distracts you from thinking about the here and now. The question is this: What do you want to happen with your alcohol or other drug use today after reflecting on the pros and cons of continuing to use them?

Useful Alcohol and Drug Facts

- Alcohol may help you to fall asleep but it causes fragmented sleep later in the night and reduces the overall quantity and healing qualities of sleep.

- Marijuana impairs attention, motor speed, and short-term memory for at least twenty-four hours after use. Most people are not aware of their impairment, making driving, for example, especially dangerous.

- Normal "safe" alcohol use is defined as no more than two drinks (one drink = one ounce of hard liquor or six ounces of wine or twelve ounces of beer) per day for men and not more than one drink a day for women.

- Drinking five or more drinks a day on a regular basis causes lasting impairment in cognitive abilities.

- Use of stimulants like cocaine or amphetamines increases the risk of stroke by causing inflammation and deterioration of the blood vessels in your brain, high blood pressure, and the clamping down of blood vessels, which can interfere with blood flow throughout your body.

Making the Change

There are many different types of changes people make that can improve their situation. Some people cut down on their use of alcohol or drugs. Others are unsure whether their use patterns are relatively safe or harmful and therefore they search for more objective information regarding their use. (Drinkers can complete a free, confidential Web-based assessment of their drinking that produces immediate personalized feedback about their drinking. See the Join Together Web site in the Resources section at the back of the book.) Some people try periods of abstinence just to try to get a better idea of what life can be like without alcohol or other drugs.

Just as there are many different types of change people can make, there are also many different ways to help change come about. Surprisingly to many, the vast majority of people with alcohol or drug use problems change completely on their own. Often health concerns, family issues, or other lifestyle changes provide an opportunity for people to reflect on their alcohol or drug use and to reevaluate the role it plays in their life. Frequently those individuals make decisions to change their use of drugs or alcohol that are successful without formal treatment, counseling, attending AA (Alcoholics Anonymous) or NA (Narcotics Anonymous), or seeking other formal help. Many people also consult their doctors about whether and how to change.

People also try AA or NA meetings, Rational Recovery, Moderation Management, or they sign up for specialized treatment. Alcohol or drug concerns are also appropriate to bring up with counselors, psychologists, social workers, clergy, or anyone else who can offer nonjudgmental support and advice. Especially for people who experience significant symptoms of dependence (e.g., craving, loss of control, compulsive use, withdrawal, blackouts) or have been unable to remain clean and sober after several serious attempts, formal treatment or support programs may be quite helpful. Often, formal treatment provides not only a break from access to alcohol or drugs, but good training in coping with abstinence and preventing relapse. AA provides a strong spiritual model and, often, tenacious social support for the person trying to recover. Clearly, there are many ways to change alcohol or other drug abuse and, hopefully, each individual will find a route best suited to him or herself.

Conclusion

The good news is that people with MS have many things they can do to improve their symptoms, their health, and their daily lives. The bad news is that it may take time, effort, support from loved ones, and sometimes support from rehabilitation or other medical professionals. Hopefully, you have identified some opportunities to improve your health, placed your progress within a stage of the change model, and planned what you can do next. Don't forget, one type of active coping is asking for help. If you get stuck, ask for help from your doctor, a rehabilitation therapist, a psychologist, or a counselor who works with people with chronic diseases such as MS.

CHAPTER 5

Managing Depression, Anxiety, and Your Emotional Challenges

Dawn M. Ehde, Ph.D. and Charles H. Bombardier, Ph.D.

HAVING MS: AN EMOTIONAL ROLLER COASTER

Living with multiple sclerosis (MS) can be very stressful. MS not only affects your physical health, it may also affect your emotional health. This disability may cause changes in your routines, your abilities, your goals, and your lifestyle. MS also can be unpredictable, which can make adapting to its changes particularly challenging. When living with MS, it is normal to feel any of a variety of emotions. At times you may feel overwhelmed, sad, angry, nervous, or worried. You may feel depressed. You may question your ability to deal with all of the changes that this disability and the treatments for it may require. At other times, you may surprise yourself and feel happy, calm, confident, and fully in control of your life. You may feel capable of handling whatever challenges MS presents you with; you may even feel grateful for some of the aspects of your life that have been changed by MS. And these are just a few of the many emotions you may feel as a result of living with MS.

In this chapter, you will learn about the various ways that MS can impact how you feel. You'll learn something about the most common emotional experiences that result from living with MS, including depression. We'll describe what depression is—and what it isn't—as it commonly appears in people with MS. You'll learn to recognize when your own emotional reactions are interfering with your life. More importantly, you'll learn skills to help you feel better and to meet the emotional challenges of MS.

Because many people not only survive but thrive following a diagnosis of MS, we will also discuss the process of bouncing back, also known as *resilience,* and we'll discuss how to build or maintain your resilience. You will have opportunities in this chapter to practice specific techniques for managing your emotional challenges.

We also want to acknowledge the fact that you may not have significant problems with your mood or emotions. Certainly, not everyone with MS experiences depression or the other emotional challenges discussed in this chapter. In fact, many individuals with MS adapt quite well to living with the chronic condition. Nonetheless, the information and skills presented in this chapter will help you to maintain your emotional health and improve your skills for managing the stress of living with MS.

It may be helpful for you to know what we mean by a few of the terms used in this chapter. When we use the word *emotions,* we are simply referring to feelings. Sadness, fear, happiness, anger, anxiety, contentment are all examples of emotions. Emotions can be *transient,* that is, temporary, or more persistent. When an emotion is all-encompassing and persistent, it is often referred to as a person's *mood.* If your mood is a persistent, negative one, you may want to change it.

COMMON EMOTIONAL EXPERIENCES

Gloria. When Gloria was diagnosed with MS, she felt very fearful. She was worried about how MS would affect her, her ability to care for her family, and her ability to work. She was afraid of what the future might hold. At times, she also felt angry that she had MS. She was also hopeful, however, that the treatments prescribed by her healthcare provider would reduce any progression of the disease and help her to keep doing everything she enjoyed doing: raising her children, nurturing her other relationships, and working.

Dan. After living with MS for more than twenty years, Dan found himself becoming moodier than usual. He noticed that he became irritated easily and was quick to lose his temper, sometimes saying things to others he later regretted. He often felt guilty after an irritable outburst or losing his temper. His family and friends were quite surprised by his outbursts because he had been known for his calm, relaxed demeanor.

Donna. It seemed that Donna was at the height of her career when she was diagnosed with MS. As the CEO of a large company, she had many responsibilities, worked long hours, and traveled a lot. She loved her job and everything that went with it. She approached her diagnosis in the same way that she approached challenges at work: with a vigorous optimism that she would meet the challenges of the disease. Sometimes she felt nervous or sad about the changes in her life, but these feelings never lasted too long and were often followed by a renewed sense of hope and optimism.

It's likely that you've experienced a number of different emotions about living with MS. You may recognize in yourself some of the feelings experienced by Gloria, Dan, and Donna. Some of the emotions may be "negative," that is, uncomfortable feelings, and some may be "positive," that is, pleasant feelings. Now, take a few minutes to think about how you've been affected by living with MS. Specifically, think about some of the emotions you've experienced and then complete the checklist that follows.

Checklist 6: Emotional Inventory

Circle the emotions that you recall feeling when you were first diagnosed with MS:

Aggravated	Depressed	Glad	Loving	Satisfied
Angry	Despair	Grouchy	Mad	Scared
Annoyed	Disappointed	Guilty	Nervous	Stressed
Anxious	Disgusted	Hope	Optimistic	Terrified
Ashamed	Edgy	Humiliated	Overwhelmed	Uneasy
Caring	Embarrassed	Hurt	Panicky	Unhappy
Compassionate	Envious	Insecure	Proud	Other:
Competent	Excited	Irritated	Rage	Other:
Courageous	Frightened	Jealous	Relieved	
Dejected	Frustrated	Lonely	Sad	

Circle the emotions that you have felt recently:

Aggravated	Dejected	Frightened	Jolly	Relieved
Amusement	Depressed	Frustrated	Joy	Sad
Angry	Despair	Glad	Jubilant	Satisfied
Annoyed	Disappointed	Grouchy	Lonely	Scared
Anxious	Disgusted	Guilty	Loving	Stressed
Ashamed	Eager	Happy	Mad	Terrified
Caring	Edgy	Hope	Nervous	Thrilled
Cheerful	Embarrassed	Humiliated	Optimistic	Triumphant
Compassionate	Enthusiastic	Hurt	Overwhelmed	Uneasy
Competent	Envious	Insecure	Panicky	Unhappy
Content	Excited	Irritated	Proud	Other:
Courageous	Exhilarated	Jealous	Rage	Other:

As always, the emotions you are currently feeling are the most important. Please take some time to describe your current emotional state as a function of the emotions you've circled. We often don't take the time to do this. This will be a kind of emotional inventory for you.

_____

_____

_____

There are several important points to understand about the emotional experiences of people with multiple sclerosis:

- Emotions can vary from person to person

- Not everyone with MS will have the same set of emotions

- Your emotions may change over time

- Emotions are neither "right" nor "wrong," and there is no "right" way to feel

- Negative emotions are not necessarily bad or destructive

- Having MS doesn't sentence you to a life of unhappiness

- People don't necessarily experience emotions in stages

- Many people with MS live happy, satisfying lives without experiencing significant depression or anxiety

- You may not be aware of "how extreme" an emotional reaction may appear to others

- Other people may project their emotional responses to MS on you

Donna. One day Donna ran into an old friend from college, Jan. Over coffee, she informed Jan about the recent events in her life, including her diagnosis of MS. After hearing of this, Jan said, "How awful! You must feel so much sadness at having that disease! You are very brave to be continuing on with your life as you are doing." Donna felt misunderstood by her friend, as well as irritated, because, in fact, she felt neither depressed nor particularly courageous. When she tried to explain this to her friend, Jan replied, "It sounds to me like you are in emotional denial about your disease. You must accept it if you are to move on with your life." This, too, irritated Donna, as she knew that she was managing her MS successfully and was living her life just the way she wanted to live.

It's important to recognize that other people in your life may expect you to have certain emotional reactions to MS. For example, when some people learn of your disease, they may assume that you feel depressed or sad about having it, regardless of how you actually feel. They may express surprise when you tell them you don't feel that way. They may overestimate the suffering caused by MS. Some may even go so far as to say you are "in denial" of your feelings.

Conversely, some people may feel very uncomfortable if you express strong emotions such as anger about having MS. They may encourage you to "always look on the bright side" and warn you that a "negative attitude" can cause you to worsen. Or they may put you on a pedestal, praising you for being "brave" or "courageous." These are just a few of the reactions you may get from others about how you are feeling about having MS. It is common for humans to make assumptions about how one should feel in response to a loss or to the presence of a disability, such as MS.

Even if such a response is well-intended, be careful not to assume that you should feel what others tell you to feel. If you are uncertain after some of these interactions as to what to do, it can be helpful to talk about them with a trusted friend, family member, or therapist. It may also be helpful to discuss this with others who have MS.

WHAT IS DEPRESSION?

Depression is the most commonly discussed emotional reaction in the MS literature. However, there can be a lot of confusion about what is meant by the term. Sometimes, the word "depression" is used to describe a temporary emotion, such as feeling sad for a couple of hours when you are having a bad day or not feeling well. Other times, the term is used to mean a pervasive mood that significantly interferes with living. This is technically called major depressive disorder (MDD), which is also sometimes referred to as "clinical depression" or simply "depression." People with MS may or may not experience depression or MDD. However, when they do, it often negatively affects all aspects of their lives. Thus, it is important to educate yourself about what MDD is, so that you can recognize it if it is present, or prevent it, in the future.

Major depression is not just feeling blue or down in the dumps. It is also more than feeling sad or experiencing grief after a loss. *Major depression* is a medical condition (just like diabetes, high blood pressure, obesity, or heart disease) that day after day affects your thoughts, feelings, physical health, and how you act. Major depression is neither your fault, nor caused by personal weakness or lack of willpower. Most importantly, there are effective treatments for major depression, which will be described later in this chapter.

Facts About Major Depression

Major depression is defined as a period of two weeks or longer in which a person experiences depressed mood or loss of pleasure most of the time, on most days, along with several other symptoms, such as significant weight changes, changes in sleep, changes in activity (either slowness or agitation), fatigue, feeling worthless or guilty, difficulty concentrating or making decisions, or thoughts of death or suicide.

Technically, to receive a diagnosis of a depressive disorder, you must have these symptoms most of the day, nearly every day, and the symptoms would need to cause significant interference with living your life. In addition to these primary symptoms, depression may cause irritability and moodiness, which can make the depressed person hard to be around. Some people who are depressed tend to want to be alone and to stay away from others. Persons who are depressed may feel hopeless and alone.

Major depressive disorder doesn't affect only those with MS. Indeed, MDD is common in the general population, affecting about one in twenty Americans each year (more than 11 million people). Almost one in four women will go through an episode of major depression sometime in her life.

People with MS are at greater risk for major depression than the general population. Approximately 25 percent of those with MS will have suffered from MDD at some point in the last year, and as many as 54 percent will suffer from it at some point in their life (Ehde and Bombardier 2005). What causes depression to occur in some, but not all, people with MS is not completely understood.

A variety of factors may contribute to the development of MDD in some people with MS. Major depressive disorder may be associated with genetics, immune dysregulation, or certain brain lesions caused by MS. Those people who have been recently diagnosed with MS, those with more severe MS disease, and those with fewer friends or social supports are more at risk for major depression (Chwastiak et al. 2002).

However, how much someone is disabled by MS doesn't necessarily determine whether that person will become depressed. For example, some people who are severely disabled by their MS do not get depressed, whereas others with MS without any disability may become depressed. Our individual capacity to deal with depression is a function of several factors, including genetics, our emotional reserves at the onset of the disability, and so forth.

Major depression may be difficult to detect because depression and MS share a number of symptoms, including fatigue, problems with concentration or memory, and changes in sleep and eating. It is also difficult to tell major depression from the normal distress associated with having a chronic, possibly progressive, illness.

The Impact of Depression

Depression is significant because it affects your ability to function in your daily life. People who are depressed may have difficulties getting things done; for example, finishing work commitments or keeping appointments. At least one study has suggested that those who are depressed are not as good at taking their MS medications as those who are not depressed (Mohr, Classen and Barrera, Jr. 2004). Depression also amplifies pain and other physical symptoms in people with chronic illnesses. Sleep problems and poor energy are characteristic of MDD and can make fatigue, already a problem for many with MS, worse. Untreated depression can last a long time, for example, from six to twelve months or more.

Josh. Josh had lived with MS for more than ten years when he suddenly began feeling very depressed, lethargic, irritable, and disinterested in life. He was quite moody, and others told him he was difficult to be around. He had difficulties falling asleep at night, and found himself not wanting to get out of bed in the morning after a night of turning and tossing and fitful sleep. Sometimes, he was so fatigued he chose to skip work and stay in bed most of the day. He didn't have much of an appetite and noticed, for the first time in his life, that he was losing weight even though he wasn't dieting. He quit swimming, which he had previously enjoyed doing. Although he had never had problems with his cognition, he began noticing he was forgetful and had difficulties concentrating when reading or working. At times, he missed his MS medications because of his forgetfulness. At other times, he chose not to take them, thinking, "Why bother?" He also observed that he was feeling more pain than usual, and he felt helpless in dealing with it. These difficulties went on for a couple months and, over time, Josh became very worried that his MS was progressing.

The first step to dealing with MDD is to recognize it. Take the self-test below as a way to determine whether any mood changes you might be experiencing may meet the criteria for MDD.

Checklist 7: The Depression Self-Test

Over the last two weeks, how often have you been bothered by any of the following problems?	Not at all	Several days	More than half the days	Nearly every day
1. Little interest or pleasure in doing things.				
2. Feeling down, depressed, or hopeless.				
3. Trouble falling or staying asleep, or sleeping too much.				
4. Feeling tired or having little energy.				
5. Poor appetite or overeating.				

6.	Feeling bad about yourself—or that you are a failure or have let yourself or your family down.			
7.	Trouble concentrating on things, such as reading the newspaper or watching television.			
8.	Moving or speaking so slowly that other people could have noticed. Or the opposite— being so fidgety or restless that you have been moving around a lot more than usual.			
9.	Thoughts that you would be better off dead or of hurting yourself in some way.			

From the Patient Health Questionnaire, ©Pfizer Inc., used with permission.

Scoring: If you checked five or more symptoms as occurring several days or more, you should probably check with your healthcare provider about whether your symptoms are due to MDD, your health, medications, or other life issues. If you checked five or more symptoms in the shaded area, your symptoms are consistent with MDD and medical attention is definitely advised. If you are experiencing thoughts of death or suicide you should notify your healthcare provider immediately, as well as others who know or care about you. The intense feelings of depression, hopelessness, or loss often leading to suicidal thoughts or actions are not permanent. These feelings and situations can be helped with medications or psychotherapy.

It's also important to point out that there are other health conditions that can cause similar symptoms. For example, if you have a thyroid problem, you may have symptoms of depression. Also, some medications can cause symptoms of depression. For example, some people who take steroids for an MS exacerbation may feel depressed. That's why it's important to talk with your healthcare provider about your symptoms, so the two of you can work together to determine what is going on and what to do.

Josh. At his family's insistence, Josh made an appointment to see his doctor about his symptoms. He was very worried his doctor would tell him that his MS was progressing. During his meeting with his doctor, they talked at length about Josh's symptoms and their impact on his life. The doctor asked Josh the same questions from the self-test you just took. After some additional questions and some medical tests to rule out any other causes, Josh's physician diagnosed Josh with MDD and recommended treatment specifically for that.

Proven Treatments for MDD

The good news is that MDD is treatable. Below, we review some of the most common treatments for MDD, mostly focusing on those that have demonstrated their effectiveness in published papers in the scientific literature. Typically, depression is treated most successfully when several strategies (pharmacologic and nonpharmacologic) are employed.

Exercise

Exercise is one of the most accessible and effective ways available to improve the quality of your life and to help with depression. Exercise is safe for people with MS and improves their fitness and strength. It is known to produce widespread positive effects in mood, quality of life, sexual functioning, recreation, pain, fatigue, and psychosocial functioning. Finally, research indicates that exercise is as effective as standard medications and psychotherapy for treating depression. Those people who exercise to treat their depression also are more likely to continue treatment and less likely to relapse into depression.

If you want to consider exercising to help your mood, it would be wise to take into account several factors. Do you have any health problems, other than MS, that might be affected by increased exercise? It would be prudent to discuss your plans to exercise with your healthcare provider before beginning any exercise program. Next, think about the types of exercise you would enjoy now or have enjoyed in the past. Common sense indicates that you'll stick with a form of exercise that you enjoy longer than you will with something not as enjoyable. Also, enjoyment may be part of the reason that makes exercise a good antidepressant for some. Finally, the type of exercise you do and even its intensity may be less important than doing something regularly; that is, doing it several times a week. So if you really like walking or Pilates but don't like aerobics classes, go with what you like.

What fits into your life and your budget? Can you fit in time to go to the gym in the morning, at lunch, after work? Would it be better to use yoga or aerobics videotapes at home? Consider "lifestyle exercise" in which you incorporate exercise into your daily life; for example, walking to work or to the store, walking up the stairs rather than taking the elevator, or even turning regular chores like vacuuming or mowing the lawn into a purposeful exercise session.

There are many good options for exercise: jogging, rowing, mall walking, swimming, treadmill training, water aerobics, Tai Chi, weight lifting, stationary biking, and martial arts. Of course, you'll want to consider individual factors such as the best time of day for you to exercise, how to keep cool during exercise, and whether you want to exercise in classes, with friends, or alone.

A measured beginning. It is usually best to start an exercise program at the low end in terms of time and intensity, and then to build yourself up gradually. For example, measure how long or far you can walk now, before you get tired. Then, set that time or distance as your initial goal. Increase the time or distance by 5 to 10 percent at each exercise outing. The principles of a classic begin-to-jog program are illustrative of a good gradual buildup for exercise. In this program, you begin jogging for only two minutes; then you walk for four minutes; repeating that cycle five times for a total of thirty minutes of exercise. You do that every other day for a week. The second week, you jog for three minutes and walk for three minutes, five times every other day. The program increases the ratio of jogging to walking gradually, until you are jogging for thirty minutes straight within ten weeks.

However you choose to begin exercising, start low, set your goals low enough so that you have a 90 percent chance of succeeding, build up gradually, and enjoy your progress. For more tips on how to start an exercise program, see chapter 4 in this workbook.

Psychotherapy

Psychotherapy can be very effective for treating depression. In fact, research suggests that psychotherapy combined with other forms of treatment, including medications, is likely the best form of treatment for MDD (Mohr, Goodkin, and Donald 1999). Psychotherapy appears to be helpful in treating depression in persons with MS, too. Cognitive behavioral therapy, as described in chapter 3, is particularly useful in treating depression. However, other psychotherapeutic approaches also can be quite effective. Whatever approach you prefer, it is important to find a therapist with whom you feel comfortable and with whom you can develop a collaborative relationship. See chapter 3 for ideas on finding a good therapist.

Medications

As evidenced by the numerous advertisements for antidepressants in today's magazines, newspapers, and commercials, there are a number of antidepressant medications that are used for treating depression. Antidepressants are thought to treat depression by altering the chemical pathways in the brain that are related to mood. Only a few studies have examined the effectiveness of antidepressant medications in treating depression in persons with MS, however. So far, it looks as if people with MS are likely to benefit from antidepressant medications, although there is no clear indication that one antidepressant is better than another for treating MS-related depression. Thus, our conclusions about medications have been drawn from what we know about treating depression in those who do not have MS.

Common antidepressants. The most common antidepressants prescribed are the selective serotonin reuptake inhibitors (SSRIs). Others include the newer antidepressants, such as the alpha-2 antagonists, selective norepinephrine reuptake inhibitors (SNRIs) and aminoketones, and the tricyclic antidepressants (TCAs). An older class of antidepressants, the monoamine oxidase inhibitors (MAOIs), are less commonly prescribed today.

Typically, antidepressant medications work gradually and require several weeks or more for their full benefit to take effect. For many antidepressants, to receive the full benefit may take six to eight weeks of treatment. **Note:** This is important because antidepressants generally will not be that quick a fix. If little or no improvement is seen after several weeks, your healthcare provider may alter the dosage of the medication, change the type of medication, or add another medication.

Typically, you will be encouraged to continue taking the medication for five months or longer, even after your depression has lifted. Some people can then discontinue the medication without experiencing any further depressive symptoms, while others who have chronic depression often benefit from staying on the medication to prevent or decrease future episodes.

Regardless of which medication you try, it's important for your health provider to closely monitor how well you are doing after you start an antidepressant course of treatment. The reason for this is that antidepressants sometimes don't work for some people, or they may not be prescribed at the right dosage, or it may not be the precisely right medication for you. It's important to inform your healthcare provider about how your depressive symptoms respond to the medication, as well as reporting any side effects. Also be sure to tell your doctor of all other medications you are taking, including any for your MS, as well as any herbal or complementary treatments, because you don't want to experience any complications that might arise because of any drug interactions.

Alternative or complementary medicines. What about the effectiveness of herbal medicines such as Saint-John's-wort and S-Adenosyl Methionine (SAM-e)? Both have received a lot of attention for their antidepressant properties. First, we recommend that you talk with your primary care physician before using other herbal or alternative medications because they can have both positive and negative effects and can interact badly with other medications you may be taking. Saint-John's-wort has been studied extensively with some studies suggesting it is helpful for mild depression; however, the best studies done so far demonstrate that it is no better than a sugar pill for people suffering from major depression (Shelton et al. 2001).

SAM-e has been studied less, but it, too, seems to improve mild depressive symptoms. SAM-e tends to improve depressive symptoms less than standard antidepressants, however (Agency for Healthcare Research and Quality 2002). When considering alternative therapies, see chapter 6 for a decision-making framework. Unfortunately, many alternative therapies that have been subjected to scientific study are of no or minimal value.

Self-Help Books

There are a number of excellent self-help books for depression. They are written primarily for people who do not have MS but they can be helpful nonetheless. *Feeling Good* by David Burns (1999) is a classic text on helping yourself overcome depression by changing how you think and act. There is also *Mind over Mood* by Dennis Greenberger and Christine Padesky (1995). Reading autobiographies of people who have struggled with depression can also be helpful. Best-selling books on this topic include *Darkness Visible* by William Styron (1990) and *The Noonday Demon* by Andrew Solomon (2001).

WHAT ABOUT ANXIETY?

Most of us have experienced anxiety at some point in our lives. For example, you may recall the feeling of butterflies in your stomach before you gave a speech, or the tension and jumpiness you felt while waiting for the results of a medical test, or the way your heart pounded after you narrowly missed being in a car accident. When anxious about an upcoming situation, you might worry, think about your concerns frequently, and have difficulties concentrating. You might have problems falling asleep the night before a big event, such as getting married or starting a new job.

In the short run, anxiety can be a normal and helpful response to situations that require us to act. It can prepare you to face a challenging or threatening situation. For example, if you are nervous before giving a speech or taking an exam, you can deal with your anxiety by practicing your speech or studying. It can be helpful to take stock of both the physical and psychological symptoms of anxiety that you're feeling by using checklist 8.

Checklist 8: Assessing Your Anxiety

Anxiety can include physical and psychological symptoms; please check (✓) those symptoms that apply to you.

Physical Symptoms	Psychological Symptoms
_____ Sweating	_____ Apprehensive
_____ Nausea	_____ Fearful
_____ Shortness of breath or rapid breathing	_____ Constant worry
_____ Heart palpitations	_____ Feeling something "bad" might happen
_____ Trembling or shaking	_____ Fear of losing control
_____ Hot flashes or chills	_____ Irritability
_____ Muscle tension or aches	_____ Uneasiness
_____ Numbness	_____ Difficulty concentrating
_____ Dizziness	_____ Thinking negatively
_____ Fatigue	_____ Feeling of terror
_____ Restlessness, feeling keyed up	_____ Fear of dying
_____ Constipation	_____ Feeling detached, unreal
_____ Diarrhea	_____ Feelings of panic

Take a few minutes to summarize the anxiety symptoms you might be feeling after you've reviewed this checklist and any others that you observe. Write a description of how you experience anxiety in the space provided below. This summary can then be discussed with your primary care physician or therapist if needed.

_____

_____

_____

_____

When you're anxious, your behavior is also affected. You may have difficulties getting things done or staying on task. Sleep can be disrupted. It is common to want to avoid whatever is making you anxious. For example, if you are really anxious about a final exam, you might decide to skip studying and go to a movie as a way to avoid your anxiety. Or you might notice that you feel detached from your relationships, tending to be preoccupied with your thoughts and worries rather than listening to others. You might find that you get irritated, anger easily, or just feel generally overwhelmed.

Melinda. On the day Melinda had an appointment with a neurologist to learn the results of her medical tests, including an MRI, she felt very nervous. Her physician had told her that she might have multiple sclerosis. She didn't know much about MS and worried it might shorten her life. She felt queasy, had difficulties sleeping the night before, and couldn't focus well enough to get any work done before her appointment. She also felt "jumpy."

Because she felt so anxious, she called a friend to ask him to accompany her to the appointment, in case the news was bad. She also went to the Internet to look up information on MS. She was relieved to see there is quite a lot of information about MS online, including some Web sites that indicate it is possible to live a happy, satisfying life even with MS. She was surprised at how much support and information there is, both on the Web and in her community to help people with MS, including the newly diagnosed. After absorbing all the new information and talking with her friend, she felt much better prepared for the news she might get from her doctor that day.

Melinda had a normal response to her situation: anxiety. It is very common to feel anxiety at the possibility of a diagnosis of MS. Many people with MS feel anxious when they learn they have it, experience exacerbations, or have to deal with the uncertainties of the disease.

Useful and Harmful Anxiety

With a new diagnosis of MS, you may worry about how much your health, your family and friends, and your ability to do what you want to do will be affected. Anxiety is an understandable and normal response to uncertain or challenging events. When anxiety prompts you to obtain help—make positive changes or fortify your coping skills and resources—it actually can be helpful. In Melinda's case, her anxiety caused her to seek information. In that way, her anxiety helped her to be better prepared for the possibility of being diagnosed with MS. When time-limited and not too intense, mild anxiety can be useful, even adaptive for everyone.

When anxiety is difficult to control, excessive, long-lasting, or disruptive to your life, it is not helpful; it may even be harmful. If you feel overwhelmed by anxiety, have many anxiety symptoms that last longer than a few weeks, or find that your anxiety is interfering with your life, you may have an anxiety disorder. Anxiety disorders, like MDD, are disorders that are likely to have a number of causes, including biological.

Anxiety disorders. Several types of anxiety disorders exist, ranging from one type in which anxiety arises only in response to a specific situation (e.g., a phobia for a needle injection) to another type, in which the anxiety is more generalized and not connected with any particular situation (free-floating anxiety). Anxiety disorders may make you feel nervous most of the time, without any apparent cause. To avoid feeling anxiety, you may stop doing certain activities.

You might even feel immobilized or terrified by your anxiety. A description of the specific types of anxiety disorders is beyond the scope of this chapter. However, for more information about the types of anxieties, as well as strategies for how to manage them, you may wish to read *The Anxiety and Phobia Workbook* by Edmund J. Bourne (2005).

Anxiety disorders are the most common of all mental disorders experienced by the general public. However, when compared to depression, less is known about the specific rates of anxiety and anxiety disorders among those with MS. Similar to depression, not everyone who has MS develops an anxiety disorder. Feelings of significant anxiety are especially common for the person with MS as well as her or his partner immediately preceding and shortly after the diagnosis of MS is made.

For those of you who are newly diagnosed, this anxiety will decrease with time. It may even motivate you to learn more about the disease, make positive changes that promote your health, fortify your resources, and plan for the future. However, if the anxiety persists or interferes with your life's activities, it may be a signal that you need to do something about it.

Injection anxiety and phobia. You may be anxious about injecting yourself with a disease-modifying medication. For some people with MS, their anxiety about self-injection causes them to avoid taking their medication or makes them unable to inject themselves. Fortunately, this type of anxiety is very responsive to a brief course of cognitive behavioral psychotherapy. If you find that you are unable to self-inject as a result of anxiety, you may wish to talk with your healthcare provider about referring you to a psychotherapist who can help you to overcome your anxiety and avoidance of self-injection.

Whether you have a full-blown anxiety disorder or more transitory anxiety, there are a number of things you can do to counter it. Occasionally, medications cause anxiety, so if you are unusually anxious, you should talk with your healthcare provider about it. Health-promoting activities such as exercise, described in this chapter as well as in chapter 4, can be useful. The other strategies described above under depression, as well as those described later in this chapter in the section on promoting resilience, are often effective in decreasing, eliminating, or managing anxiety. If you think you have a full-blown anxiety disorder, you may wish to see a therapist. (See chapter 3 for tips on finding a therapist.)

Psychotherapy, particularly cognitive behavioral psychotherapy, is an effective treatment for anxiety disorders. In addition, a number of medications can be useful in treating anxiety. You may wish to talk with your healthcare provider or a psychiatrist about medications for anxiety. In most cases, mild anxiety can be addressed through the strategies described in this chapter as well as through psychotherapy. For moderate to severe anxiety disorders, a combination of medication and psychotherapy may be indicated. For a few types of anxiety, including phobias, psychotherapy (often cognitive behavioral) is the first line of approach to treatment.

IRRITABILITY AND MOODINESS

People with MS sometimes describe feeling irritable, cranky, or easily frustrated more often than they were before being diagnosed with MS. Irritability can be a symptom of other emotional challenges, such as depression, anxiety, or stress. It also can be caused by other difficulties such as sleep problems, pain, fatigue, or cognitive difficulties. For some, changes in how the brain regulates moods also can contribute to irritability.

If you find yourself feeling cranky or irritable more than you like, notice when you start feeling irritable. You may wish to write down what is going on at the time you are feeling irritable. You may notice patterns to your irritability that will help you figure out what to do.

For example, have you noticed that you get irritable at the end of the day, when you are feeling tired? You might also be irritable when you are anxious or simply when you are overstimulated. If you don't notice a pattern to your irritability but do notice that you feel irritable much of the time, you should consider talking with a healthcare provider. Your irritability may be the result of a major depressive disorder, for example, or a side effect of one of your steroid medications. Psychotherapy can be helpful in recognizing contributors to irritability and in learning ways to manage it.

Brain changes. Sometimes, changes in the brain associated with MS also can lead to difficulty in controlling your emotions, for example, controlling your mood or visible displays of your emotions. In such instances, a person may be perceived as moody or as showing emotions that seem out of character or unsuitable for the situation. For example, if you have this syndrome, you may cry more easily, or be quick to become angry or upset. You may laugh at a time that seems inappropriate for the situation.

If you notice these difficulties in controlling your emotions, or others have described observing such emotions in you, this may be due to your MS. If such emotional changes interfere with your relationships, your activities, your work, or your self-esteem, you should consider learning more about them as well as finding ways to decrease such emotional control challenges.

Talk with your healthcare provider, as well as to others with MS. They may help you better understand how your emotions sometimes can be dysregulated by neurological changes. They may also recommend psychotherapy or medications that can help to regulate your moods better. When the difficulty in controlling emotions is extreme, sometimes certain medications can be helpful.

BUILDING RESILIENCE

As mentioned earlier in this chapter, not every emotion experienced in MS is negative. In fact, many people find that they are able to meet the challenges of living with MS successfully, and to live happy, satisfying lives. People who "bounce back" from difficulties are sometimes described as having "resilience." This topic is just as important, if not more, than knowing about depression, because it holds the key to managing the challenges and emotions that can accompany MS.

Before we describe what we mean by resilience, please do the following exercise as it can help to better ground this concept for you.

WORKSHEET 13:   INVENTORY OF YOUR PERSONAL STRENGTHS

What do you know about your own abilities to cope with the challenges of MS? Please take a few minutes to think about the personal strengths that aid you in managing your emotions. Then, write them down in the space provided below. Answering the following questions will help you to identify some of the strengths and strategies you already possess.

What are some things you have accomplished while living with MS? *Examples:* Successfully raised children, developed a new hobby, worked part-time at the local bookstore, and so on.

_____

_____

_____

What has helped you meet the challenges of life, including MS? These might be personal characteristics, such as qualities or skills you have, or they may be things you do (your own actions). *Examples:* Am a positive thinker, maintain my sense of humor, or listen to upbeat music, and so on.

_____

_____

_____

List people you can turn to for assistance or support, emotional or practical. *Examples:* My spouse, my MS support group, my friends with whom I volunteer at the food bank, and so on.

_____

_____

_____

What other strengths or support do you have that you can tap? *Examples:* My faith, my church or temple, my next-door neighbor, and so on.

_____

_____

_____

What did you learn from doing this exercise? Hopefully, this helped you to see some of the strengths you have more clearly. Sometimes, we tend to focus on the problems or challenges of MS. We lose sight of all the good things that we experience or become "in spite of" or sometimes even "because of" the challenges of living with MS.

This process of adapting well to or bouncing back from significant challenges is known as *resilience.* Being resilient doesn't mean that you don't experience discouragement or emotional distress. Such experiences are common and may be part of the resilience process itself.

When you are resilient, you experience such feelings but you don't let those feelings define who you are or how you respond to challenges.

The remainder of this chapter will focus on how to learn, nurture, and practice resilience. The skills that follow will not only help you build or maintain resilience, they will also help you to decrease stress, anxiety, and other negative emotions that you may experience.

Strategies to Cultivate Resilience and Manage Your Emotions

Research in the fields of health and psychology has shown that a number of skills are very useful for building resilience and positive mood, reducing stress, treating depression, and promoting health. These skills include some of the matters discussed in other chapters, including chapter 4 on health promotion and chapter 13 on spirituality. The main skills for cultivating resilience and promoting healthy emotions fall into the following categories:

1. Nurturing positive emotions. Look for them, focus on them, create them.

2. Getting active, physically and socially.

3. Practicing relaxation skills.

4. Thinking differently about challenges.

5. Using support from others.

Nurturing Positive Emotions

Positive emotions play a very important role in our health. By "positive emotions" we mean experiencing feelings that make you feel good; for example, feeling joy, happiness, laughter, playful. So, when we say "positive emotions," we are talking about "feeling good" emotionally.

As you probably know from your own life, positive emotions such as joy, laughter, and contentment can and do occur even in the face of difficulties, such as a recent loss, disability, or adversity. For example, after a difficult board meeting, a "frazzled" businesswoman looks forward joyfully to spending the evening at home with her spouse and family. And it is common at memorial services to laugh when recalling humorous events that involved the deceased.

It is a good idea to try to have positive emotions on a daily basis. Experiencing positive emotions during a stressful or difficult time can be particularly helpful, for a number of reasons. Positive emotions can:

- Increase creativity

- Decrease distress

- Increase flexibility of attitude and thinking

- Prevent depression, chronic stress, and anxiety

- Help with problem solving

- Serve as a break from stress

- Improve physical health

So, how can you increase positive emotions in your daily life when you need to? You may not realize it, but you probably do things every day that cause you to feel good, even if for just a few minutes. For example, do you read the comics? Listen to certain CDs? Watch sit-coms? Snuggle with your cat? Share jokes with your child? Laugh with the counterperson at the coffee shop or grocery store? There are many things we can do to help us feel good emotionally.

Now, turn to worksheet 14 on building positive experiences. Take a few minutes to list some things you have found help you feel good (emotionally).

WORKSHEET 14:   BUILDING POSITIVE EXPERIENCES

Things I currently do that make me feel good (emotionally):

_____

_____

Now, take a few moments to write down some things you really want to do to build more positive emotions into your life. This can be a combination of things you are doing already and things you haven't tried. They may be simple things that don't take a lot of time, like singing in the shower, listening to your favorite music in the car, or spending a few minutes cuddling with your pet. They may be things that require a little more time, such as hobbies, recreational pursuits, exercise, relaxation exercises, or other activities. They may involve other people, such as talking to a friend, volunteering, or spending more time with a family member.

If you have a hard time coming up with ideas, talk to a friend or family member for their ideas. You already may be doing or using some things that make you feel more positive without realizing it. If you are at a loss for ideas, review the entertainment section of your newspaper for amusing and inexpensive activities or cultural events, or call the closest tourist office in your area. These "pleasant events" can take planning and involve more of your time. But the investment in time and planning will be worth it.

Things I can do to make me feel good in the future (may require some planning):

_____

_____

_____

Get Active

One of the best ways for you to improve or maintain your health, physical and emotional, is to exercise. Take a moment to focus on exercise. Exercise is certainly an important part of being active and healthy. It is an important potential treatment for people with MS. Physical activity may include a number of things. Please check those that you'd like to consider learning and those that you know and continue to do:

_____ Aerobic classes	_____ Climbing stairs	_____ Hiking
_____ Strength training	_____ Gardening	_____ Household chores
_____ Water aerobics/exercise	_____ Floor exercises	_____ Stretching
_____ Swimming	_____ Jogging or jog/walk	_____ Sedentary exercises
_____ Yoga	_____ Weight training	_____ Horseback riding
_____ Cycling	_____ Parking further from the store to walk	
_____ Racquet sports (tennis, racquetball, badminton)		_____ Other

An important point to remember is to exercise within your tolerance limits. Your doctor and physical therapist can help you to figure out what your limits are and which of your desired exercises might be best for you. Exercise, however, will build tolerance. Exercise within a group context is physically positive while also providing a social, "mood-elevating" experience.

You can use the information in chapter 4 to help you set realistic goals for incorporating more physical activity into your life. If you think that you could benefit from more activity, set a goal of increasing your activity in the next week. You may wish to set reasonable exercise goals (e.g., beginning with just a few minutes a day), increasing gradually, from week to week or month to month. You also may get ideas on exercising with MS from national or local MS organizations as well as from the Internet.

Relax

Relaxation strategies are techniques that can promote feelings of well-being, relaxation, and calmness. There are a number of ways you can try to achieve the " relaxation response," which is a physical state of deep comfort and rest that has a number of positive physiological changes associated with it, including decreased blood pressure and muscle tension. Learning to relax your body and mind can have positive effects for your physical and emotional health. Some of these strategies involve deep breathing others involve imagining peaceful images or scenery.

Whatever the technique, regular use of relaxation strategies are likely to help you feel better and may also benefit other MS symptoms, such as pain or fatigue. If you are interested in learning specific relaxation techniques, you may wish to obtain the *Relaxation and Stress Reduction Workbook* (Davis, Eschelman, and McKay 2000). There are also a number of useful tapes or CDs available that can teach you how to relax. You may wish to check out the relaxation tapes available through the Mind/Body Medical Institute (see the Web site address in the Resources section at the back of the book).

Think Differently

The way we talk to ourselves is called *self-talk*. When we refer to "self-talk," we are referring to how we think or the things that we say to ourselves. Our self-talk influences how we feel, including our moods and our pain, both physical and emotional. Holding an internal dialogue is quite normal. It can be helpful, if your self-talk is positive, or unhelpful, if it is negative. Your inner conversations have a powerful impact on how you feel.

For example, let's take a look at a common situation: being stuck in traffic. Let's say you get stuck in traffic on your way to a doctor's appointment. If you think to yourself, "This is terrible. I'm stuck and going to be really late! I'll never get to my appointment on time! My doctor will be angry with me! What an idiot I am for picking this route. I should have known there would be traffic!," what do you think you might feel while you are saying these things to yourself? You are right. You are likely to feel bad: anxious, stressed, angry, frustrated, and so forth.

Now, let's say you are in the same situation, stuck in traffic, and you say to yourself: "They must be working on the road. Sometimes things don't work as planned. Oh well, it looks like I'm going to be here for a while, so I might as well call ahead and let them know I will be late. Guess it gives me some time to listen to my new CD, or a radio show, or simply to be quiet." What do you think you might feel if you said this to yourself? You still will be late and you might feel mildly anxious or annoyed, but you won't be so worked up about it, and your feelings will be more in accord with the situation.

If you think negative or alarming thoughts, you tend to feel bad. If you think positive or reassuring thoughts, you tend to feel good or, in difficult situations, better. When you feel bad, which can mean angry, depressed, irritable, anxious, and so forth, it is usually because you've had negative or alarming thoughts, like cognitive "sinkholes." So what can you do to feel better? Basically, change how you think. If you change your thought, you'll change your feeling. It sounds simple, but it can take some practice. In fact, there are a few steps to help you change the thought.

Step 1: Become aware of your negative self-talk. Becoming aware of exactly what you are saying to yourself can help you understand why you react the way you do to events and people in your life. Self-talk is so automatic and subtle that often you don't notice it or the effect it has on your mood. You react without noticing what you told yourself right before you reacted.

It's important to step back and see the connection between what you say to yourself and how you react to situations. One way to become more aware of self-talk is to work backwards. When you notice yourself experiencing a strong emotion (e.g., anger, depression, guilt, joy), ask yourself what is occurring. What is the situation? And then ask yourself what you are saying to yourself about the situation. What thoughts are running through your head? Identify your negative self-talk. What do you say to yourself when you are sad, angry, or depressed?

Look at the table below and read the example. Then, in the space provided below the example, try to come up with three examples of your own negative self-talk.

My Negative Self-Talk		
Emotions	What is occurring	My self-talk
Example: Guilt	Not able to go to my daughter's ballgame due to fatigue	"I am a lousy parent." "I should go to her game, even if I am fatigued." "Why won't I push myself?"

Step 2: Change your negative self-talk. The most effective way to change negative self-talk is to get rid of it. When you catch yourself thinking negatively, just stop it. You may find it helpful to imagine a stop sign, which can serve to remind you to "stop" your negative thinking. Reframe your thoughts with more helpful, realistic self-talk. *Countering* involves writing down and rehearsing more accurate and functional thoughts. It's a form of mental reprogramming. Sometimes this comes easily; other times it takes some practice.

One more thing you can do to change how you think is to fill your mind with positive, reassuring, and humorous thoughts as much as possible. What are some things you can tell yourself to help you feel better and manage the challenges of living with MS (or living, in general, for that matter)? In the space provided in the table below, write down some of your common negative thoughts on the left side, and then write down your positive thoughts to counteract your negative thoughts on the right side.

My negative self-talk	More positive self-talk
Example: "I am useless. I can't work as hard or as long as I used to."	"I am doing the best I can do." "I may not work as many hours, but I have a lot of useful experience to contribute to the success of the mission."

If you find that you tend to think negatively a lot of the time, you may wish to read more on this topic. See the section Talking Yourself Through Challenges below for more ideas. You may want to use another workbook that discusses in greater detail how to change negative thinking; *Thoughts & Feelings: Taking Control of Your Moods and Your Life* is an excellent workbook (McKay, Davis, Fanning 1997). You may also find it helpful to talk to a therapist, especially one who specializes in cognitive behavioral treatment, as this approach specifically targets the negative thoughts that make you feel bad.

You can also try to experience and look for more humor in your life. Humor can be an effective strategy for dealing with stressful life events.

Humor helps us to:

- avoid jumping to negative conclusions

- avoid blowing things out of proportion

- make more balanced and reasonable assessments of our problems

- enjoy positive moments

- have a favorable impact on those around us

- increase our support and cooperation from others

Talking Yourself Through Challenges

We all have the ability to talk to ourselves. In fact, we often carry on a running conversation with ourselves throughout the day. Whether we talk to ourselves aloud or silently, we can use this ability to coach ourselves through difficult challenges. Although you already talk to yourself during difficult situations, you may not always be aware of this process. That's why many of the internal conversations we have with ourselves are referred to as "automatic self-talk." It occurs automatically, without much awareness on our part.

Here are some steps to help you talk yourself through difficult challenges.

Prepare for the challenge. You can prepare for a challenge by talking to yourself in a way that will increase your feelings of control over the situation. You need to think in terms of how you'll deal with it, and what you'll gain from this experience, even though it may be stressful. You need to stop yourself from blowing things out of proportion and suffering before the challenge really takes place.

It often helps to make a list of useful statements to say to yourself when you are preparing for the challenge. You can say things like:

"It won't help matters to sit and worry about it." "It might not be fun, but I can handle it."

"I'll use my problem-solving skills to make a plan." "Some anxiety helps performance."

You can also prepare for a challenge by going over what it will be like in your mind. Visualize yourself going through the situation while using your problem-solving skills when things become stressful.

Confront the challenge. Tell yourself that you are someone who knows how to use coping skills effectively. Learn how to talk yourself through the challenge. Use your creativity to think of things you can say to yourself when you are confronted by challenging situations. Be willing to make mistakes. Don't force yourself to be perfect. Say to yourself statements like these:

"This is tough, but I will survive." "Relax, I must concentrate on what I have to do."

"Stick to my plan. Don't get negative." "If I act as if I'm in control, I will feel that way."

Reflect on what you've learned. When the challenge is over, you should take some time to reflect on what you learned. It's okay to notice your mistakes and ask yourself how you can improve, so long as you are not too critical. You need to be willing to look at new ways of doing things. But you must also be sure to look at what you did right. When the challenge has ended, say to yourself things like this:

"It wasn't as bad as I expected." "I did pretty well and I can do even better next time."

"Life is full of difficult challenges. I might as well learn how to cope with them."

Seek Support from Others

Another strategy to build resilience and cope with difficult emotions is to seek support from others. There are a number of ways you can do this. It can be as simple as talking to a supportive family member or friend. You can also seek out more formal support, through MS support group meetings, telephone networks, Web-based discussion groups, church groups, or therapy. You can join a social group, such as a book club, hobby association, historical or arts group, or a volunteer organization as ways to find and receive more informal support.

Conclusion

So, how can you put all of this together to help yourself feel better? You might try thinking about your life as if it were a car. Sometimes, when your car breaks down because of the stress and strain of doing what cars do, you just need one part to fix it and get it running again. Other times, you may need a mechanic and several new parts before it can be fixed.

The same is true for using the skills we've been discussing in this chapter. Sometimes, when we are in stressful situations, using one skill ("part"), for example, thinking differently, relaxing, or exercising can do the trick to get us bouncing back and feeling better. Other times, it may take several kinds of techniques to feel better. If you are feeling really sad, depressed, anxious, or angry, you may wish to consult a mental health "mechanic"; that is, a therapist or your physician (see chapter 3). Whatever your situation, we hope that you recognize you have many strengths and tools to assist you in managing any emotional challenges presented by your MS.

CHAPTER 6

Alternative Therapy Considerations

Allen C. Bolwling, MD, Ph.D.

RESOLVING ALTERNATIVE (COMPLEMENTARY) MEDICINE CONFUSION

In the United States and other countries, alternative medicine use is quite popular. For people with chronic diseases, such as multiple sclerosis (MS), the use of these unconventional therapies appears to be especially common. If you have MS and are interested in determining whether a particular unconventional therapy is worth using, it can be confusing, frustrating, and time-consuming. There is so much information given to you in support groups, Web chat rooms, and so forth. How do you make sense of and evaluate all this information? To start, read this chapter. It will provide you with background information and approaches that will help you be thoughtful and careful in your evaluations of specific alternative therapies.

WHAT IS "ALTERNATIVE MEDICINE"?

The question posed above is surprisingly hard to answer. Part of the difficulty is that there are many different terms used to describe this area. In addition to "alternative medicine," other commonly used terms are "complementary medicine," "unconventional medicine," and "integrative medicine."

The broadest of these terms is *unconventional medicine*. This is often defined as those therapies that are not typically taught in medical schools or generally available in hospitals. However, this definition is unusual in that it states what unconventional medicine is not, as opposed to what it is. Also, most American medical schools now have at least limited coursework in unconventional medicine. A more complex but precise definition is that provided by the National Institutes of Health (NIH). This definition divides unconventional medicine into subcategories. The subcategories, with representative examples, are as follows:

- Biologically-based therapies (diets, dietary supplements)

- Mind-body therapies (guided imagery, meditation, stress prevention)

- Alternative medical systems (traditional Chinese medicine, homeopathy)

- Manipulative and body-based therapies (chiropractic, reflexology, massage, acupuncture)

- Energy therapies (therapeutic touch, magnets)

- Lifestyle and disease prevention (exercise, diet, sleep)

Several of the other terms used in this area are based on the way in which these unconventional therapies are used. *Alternative medicine* refers to unconventional therapies that are used instead of conventional medicine, while *complementary medicine* refers to the use of these therapies in conjunction with conventional medicine. A broader term is *complementary and alternative medicine*. In this chapter, CAM, an acronym for *complementary and alternative medicine,* is used. The combined use of unconventional and conventional medicine is known as *integrative medicine*.

IF YOU ARE INTERESTED IN ALTERNATIVE MEDICINE, YOU ARE NOT ALONE

Several studies have evaluated the use of CAM in the general population and in people with MS. According to one large survey of the general population in the United States, about 40 percent of people use some form of unconventional therapy. This survey found that people actually visited unconventional medical practitioners more frequently than primary care physicians. Nearly 20 percent of those surveyed were taking some type of herb or vitamin in addition to their prescription medications. Almost half of those surveyed were using CAM without the advice of a physician or unconventional medical practitioner, and more than half (60 percent) did not discuss their use of CAM with their personal physician (Eisenberg et al. 1998).

Studies indicate that CAM use is more common among people with MS than in the general population. One-half to two-thirds of people with MS have used some form of unconventional therapy (Bowling and Stewart 2003). The majority of you with MS are mid-career at the onset of disability, well-educated, and open to exploring options. Interestingly, people with MS usually use the phrase "unconventional medicine" along with "conventional medicine." In other words, the term is nearly always used in a complementary fashion. Only a very small fraction of you with MS use "unconventional medicine" instead of "conventional medicine" (Bowling and Stewart 2003). The CAM therapies used most commonly by people with MS include diets, dietary supplements, prayer and spiritual practices, chiropractic medicine, and massage.

THE QUALITY OF ALTERNATIVE MEDICINE INFORMATION VARIES

If you've tried to research some kind of CAM therapy, you've probably found that it can be difficult to find reliable information. There are a variety of information sources, but all of these sources have limitations.

Books

Books are one possible source of information. To evaluate the quality of information about MS found in books about alternative medicine, we conducted a survey with the Rocky Mountain MS Center (Bowling, Ibrahim, and Stewart 2000). Examining the stock of two large bookstores, we reviewed the sections on MS in fifty different alternative medicine books. In these books, MS was sometimes incorrectly defined as a form of muscular dystrophy, five to six different therapies were generally recommended, and no two books carried the same recommendations. Furthermore, it was rare for any CAM therapy to be discouraged and, sometimes, dangerous therapies were actually recommended. Given this type of information, it's easy to see how you can become very confused and, after reading a few books, you can wind up with a list of fifteen to twenty different CAM therapies for treating MS.

Other Information Sources

Other information sources also have limitations. The Internet has variable quality CAM information, particularly the chat room information. Vendors of products, such as dietary supplements, and providers of CAM services may have limited MS-specific information or exaggerate claims about the effectiveness of their products. Finally, conventional health providers, almost by definition, have limited CAM knowledge and experience.

WHAT CAN YOU DO?

Given these limitations in CAM information, you can really feel "at a loss" as people make different recommendations. There are several strategies, however, that can be very helpful. They are as follows:

- Develop a knowledge base and a set of skills that will help you assess CAM therapies.

- Take a thoughtful approach to using CAM therapies.

- Know what sources of CAM information are reliable.

The remainder of this chapter will focus on helping you to develop the strategies discussed above.

Using Evidence to Evaluate Therapies

It is extremely important for you to know the different types of evidence that may be available about the safety and effectiveness of a particular therapy. This type of evidence applies to conventional medicine as well as to unconventional medicine.

Theory

Theory is the least reliable information about any given therapy. An example of a theoretical argument about a CAM therapy for MS would be that a certain dietary supplement, "Compound X," is thought to suppress the immune system because its chemical structure is similar to another chemical that suppresses the immune system. Since suppressing the immune system may be therapeutic for some people with MS, it theoretically could be argued that Compound X may be helpful for MS. The problem with this type of information is that it is pure theory. If the compound were actually to be tested, it might be found that it does not, in fact, suppress the immune system and has no effect whatsoever on people with MS.

Experimental Evidence

Information established by experimental evidence is more reliable than theory, but it still has significant limitations. In terms of MS therapies, experimental evidence often involves studies of the effects of a therapy on the immune system and on animals with an MS-like disease known as EAE (experimental allergic encephalomyelitis).

In the case of Compound X, experimental evidence might be test-tube experiments showing that Compound X does inhibit certain components of the immune system and that it does have therapeutic effects in the animal model of MS. But this type of information still has potential problems. It could be that, in spite of the experimental evidence, actual testing of the compound on people like yourself would show that it has no effect. In fact, there is a long list of potential MS therapies that looked very promising in experimental studies but proved to be ineffective for treating the disease. Most importantly, some of these promising therapies actually ended up worsening the disease. For this reason, clinical evidence is essential.

Clinical Trial Evidence

Clinical evidence is the highest quality evidence. The best type of clinical evidence is obtained through studies known as multi-center, randomized, double-blind, placebo-controlled clinical trials. This can sound intimidating, but what this would mean in the case of Compound X is that a large number of people were randomly chosen to receive a placebo or Compound X (randomized, placebo-controlled). The patients and the clinical staff did not know who received the placebo or Compound X (double-blind), and the study was carried out at multiple institutions (multi-center). If people treated with Compound X fared significantly better than those who were on the placebo, then this is the strongest evidence that Compound X is an effective therapy.

Conducting formal clinical trials is very expensive, especially in the field of MS. For studies of CAM therapies, high levels of research funding are not readily available. Consequently, if you are interested in exploring CAM, it may be necessary for you to gamble with the information that is available. In such a situation, it may be most reasonable for you to consider therapies that are possibly effective and have very little associated risk.

It is important to recognize that the best clinical evidence that is available for altering the course of MS is that of the FDA-approved MS medications, which include interferon beta-1a (Avonex, Rebif), interferon beta-1b (Betaseron), glatiramer acetate (Copaxone), and mitoxantrone (Novantrone). If you have MS, you should strongly consider these medications, regardless of your interest in CAM therapies.

Theoretical or Experimental Evidence Is Not Clinical Evidence

Some CAM literature confuses the various levels of evidence or makes strong recommendations on the basis of relatively weak evidence. For example, you might read that a CAM therapy is highly recommended for MS because it suppresses the immune system, produces beneficial effects in the animal model of MS, and has very few side effects. At first glance, that might seem convincing. However, as noted above, all of that may be true but, unfortunately, it is still quite likely that this therapy would not be an effective treatment for MS.

When Is It Reasonable to Use Unconventional Therapies?

If you are interested in CAM, it's important to have a sense for when it may be appropriate to consider using CAM therapies. If you have a symptom that is relatively mild, such as a low level of fatigue or muscle stiffness, then it may be reasonable to use CAM. Moreover, if you have a condition for which conventional medicine has no effective therapies or only partially effective therapies, then it may be reasonable to use CAM.

On the other hand, there are some symptoms for which CAM should not be used or should be used only with caution. For example, severe conditions, such as intense pain or disabling muscle stiffness, should not be treated exclusively with unconventional therapies. However, in these situations, it may be reasonable to use conventional medicine along with CAM.

Checklist 9: Your Plan in Considering a CAM Therapy

If you are considering a CAM therapy, there are specific steps that should be taken. Please review those steps below.

Have you:

_____ Considered all of the possible conventional and CAM therapies?

_____ Assessed why you want to use a particular CAM therapy?

_____ Secured reliable information about the safety, effectiveness, cost, and effort involved?

Note: Therapies worth considering are those that don't involve a large amount of effort and are possibly effective, probably safe, and of low to moderate cost.

_____ Discussed it with your physician or other conventional health care provider?

_____ Monitored the therapy for a response, and discontinued its use if it produced side effects or was not effective?

Use caution. For most CAM therapies, information about safety and effectiveness is incomplete. As a result, there is some risk-taking involved with many forms of CAM. With an informed and careful decision-making process, however, this risk can be minimized and reasonable gambles can be made.

Watch Out for the "Warning Signs" of Questionable Therapies

There are some aspects of CAM therapies that should raise your suspicions. These "red flags" include the following:

- Little or no unbiased information available about safety or effectiveness

- "Secret ingredients" (this is always a glaring signal)

- Excessively strong claims about effectiveness

- Claims that a single therapy is effective for many different diseases

- Heavy use of "testimonials" in which very strong claims are made by individuals who claim to have used the product or service

- Much effort is involved, such as inpatient treatment, intravenous therapy, or injections

- Information about a therapy conveys a strong antiscience or anti–conventional medicine feeling

Be Aware of Myths About Dietary Supplements

In the area of dietary supplements, there are many myths, some of which are perpetuated by dietary supplement vendors. These myths include the following:

- Some supplements are claimed to have therapeutic effects and absolutely no side effects. This is not a realistic situation. Dietary supplements, like medications, contain chemicals that may be therapeutic but may also be toxic.

- More may not be better. It is sometimes claimed that if a low dose of a supplement is beneficial, then a high dose must be even better. This is not true and may be dangerous. For many supplements, high doses actually may produce side effects.

- "Natural" compounds may not be safe. There are claims that products that are natural must be safe and beneficial. This is certainly not true. There are many different natural products that are quite toxic, such as mercury, arsenic, poisonous plants, and animal venoms.

Remember That MS Involves Excessive Immune System Activity

Some alternative medicine books make an error about MS. In these books, it is stated that MS is a disease of the immune system, and that, as a result, you should take dietary supplements that stimulate your immune system. This may then be followed by a recommendation that you should take five to ten different dietary supplements to activate your immune system. **Note:** This is incorrect and is potentially dangerous! MS is an immune system disease, but it is characterized by *too much*, not too little, immune system activity. Consequently, effective MS therapies generally decrease the activity of the immune system.

In a related way, you should be wary of therapies that are claimed to be effective for MS as well as for cancer and AIDS. The treatment goals are usually the opposite in these diseases. In MS we try to decrease the immune system activity, while in AIDS and cancer we try to stimulate the immune system.

WHERE YOU CAN GET MORE INFORMATION ABOUT CAM

In addition to using the guidelines and approaches recommended in this chapter, it is important to have resources to go to for information about specific therapies. To assist people with MS in this process, the Rocky Mountain MS Center has established the Complementary and Alternative Medicine Program. One of the major aims of this program is to provide user-friendly, objective, MS-relevant CAM information. Much of this information can be accessed through this program's Web site (ms-cam.org/CAMbanner. htm), or that of the National Multiple Sclerosis Society (www.nationalmssociety.org/spotlight=cam.asp). Through the Complementary and Alternative Medicine Program, this chapter's author (Dr. Bowling) has published a book, *Alternative Medicine and Multiple Sclerosis,* with objective data on the most popular complementary or alternative medicines being used or discussed. Other information is available through the Web site of the National Multiple Sclerosis Society.

Conclusion

CAM can be both confusing and controversial. At the same time, for some people with MS, CAM may be an important component of an individualized treatment plan. Using CAM may provide many benefits, including therapeutic effects, hope, and a sense of control. Using the guidelines and approaches outlined in this chapter and the information referenced elsewhere should allow you to pursue CAM in a safe and effective manner.

CHAPTER 7

Employment Strategies and Community Resources

Robert T. Fraser, Ph.D., C.R.C.

As someone with multiple sclerosis (MS), you face a number of employment challenges within your community with the onset of this disability. Typically, onset occurs sometime in the thirties or forties when you are deeply involved in your career. Consequently, there are a number of immediate concerns that can leap out at you. These concerns can take the form of these questions: "Can I continue to work, particularly in my challenging/stressful field?" "Will I become too fatigued over the workday to continue at my job?" "Can I focus and cognitively complete my major work functions?" "Maybe I should change jobs?" "How should I go about it?" "Should I work part-time and/or consider Social Security Disability Income (SSDI)?" "Maybe I can use the Family Medical Leave Act (FMLA) to reduce my work hours or take time off?" "Could I be self-employed or possibly work at home?" "What resources are available to me in the community?" "In general, what are my options?"

These types of questions can overwhelm you at the time of your initial diagnosis and as you experience the disability and try to adapt to it. In this chapter, the full range of these issues will be addressed.

STAYING ON THE JOB

If you are newly diagnosed and your medications are new or being adjusted, it is important to utilize the Family Medical Leave Act (FMLA). Information from your physician is kept separately from your personnel file and you are not required to disclose your disability to your superior or to your coworkers. The twelve weeks of permitted time off do not have to be taken in one segment. Furthermore, the actual hours taken from work can be spread out so that you leave work for as few as one to two hours early every day, because that is all you can physically or cognitively handle. Be creative with this time and be sure to contact your company's Personnel/Human Resources or Disability Services department. That department will have specialists on the provisions of the act (FMLA).

Family Medical Leave Act (FMLA)

This act is a federal law that enables you to use up to twelve weeks of nonpaid medical leave over the course of twelve months due to your MS. Again, it can be used all at once, or it can be spread out over a year. Your spouse, biological parent, son, or daughter can also use it to provide for your care and independent living assistance (e.g., shopping, cooking, etc.) while you are receiving treatment. FMLA payments cover both private and publicly held companies with fifty or more workers. You must have been employed for 1,250 hours during the year before you become eligible for this leave. Certain key personnel within companies may be excluded from FMLA coverage. You will again need to check with your company's specialists. For further information, contact your local office of the U.S. Department of Labor. Some states also offer this leave to family members. Check the federal government pages in your phone book for the number of your state's Department of Labor.

Disclosure

If you have a good relationship with your employer, a clear disclosure of your disability with an explanation of your functional limitations can be very important. When you do this disclosure, however, it is critical to research (to the best of your abilities) the best work accommodations specific to your limitations. See chapter 8 for the procedure for examining your accommodation needs and consultation services.

This procedure could involve reviewing the Work Experience Survey (WES developed by Dr. Richard Roessler and colleagues at the Arkansas Rehabilitation Research and Training Center [see appendix A for the survey]). It could also involve spending some time with a rehabilitation counselor or assistive technologist.

Work accommodations can be procedural (a modification of how things are done), involve some structural changes to your workstation or moving your workstation (e.g., closer to a building entrance or to restroom facilities), or the use of some type of assistive technology (e.g., specialized software, such as voice-activated software).

Practice Your Disability Disclosure

You should carefully practice your actual disclosure statement. Your statement should be relatively free of medical jargon, focused on the limitations and specific accommodations that you are seeking, and brief but concise. If you present this information in a clear and positive manner to your employer, he or she will feel a significant amount of reassurance and be inclined to better engage in the process. You do not have to disclose MS, but, basically, you do need to describe "a disability" that presents certain limitations. See the National Multiple Sclerosis Society Web site in the Resources section at the back of the book for a more detailed discussion of disclosure with practice (e.g., role-play with a friend). Note that role-play can make the disclosure a much easier process to go through.

WORKSHEET 15:   DEVELOP YOUR DISCLOSURE SCRIPT

Example

Thanks for meeting with me, Ms. Kindress. I've really enjoyed working here in the accounting department. However, I need to bring to your attention the fact that I now have a disability which causes me to get tired in the early afternoon. (Disclose the actual disability at your discretion.) I feel that I can continue to do my job well if you can make an accommodation in my work hours. Such an accommodation would be in my best interests and that of the company. I would like to come in earlier by an hour and take a two-hour rest in my office between 12 and 2 P.M. In this way, I know I can maintain my proficiency over time and continue to be an asset to the company.

My Script

I need to bring to your attention the fact that I now have a disability which [describe functional limitation] _____

_____

_____

I feel that I can continue to do my job, but an accommodation is in my best interests and that of the company. I would benefit from [describe accommodation] _____

_____

_____

If a local accommodations consultant is needed and one is not available, or the company cannot find technical assistance (as mandated by the Americans with Disabilities Act [ADA]), resources such as West Virginia University's Job Accommodation Network (JAN) can be utilized (see Resources). See also see the material on accommodations in chapter 8.

ASSISTANCE FROM A STATE VOCATIONAL REHABILITATION AGENCY

Every state in the United States has a state vocational rehabilitation agency that is funded by a federal-state dollar match. Usually, as a person with MS, you will fit the level one category of eligibility under an *order of selection* based upon MS being considered a severe disability. This will all be explained to you when you visit your local agency (found in the phone book's state agency listings) during orientation to the program. A state agency rehabilitation counselor and/or consultant can help you keep your job by tapping the accommodation resources that will work best for you. If it is determined that you cannot be accommodated and there is not another reassignment job possibility within your company, then you would become eligible for the full gamut of vocational services that your state provides.

The state vocational rehabilitation agency can pay for or conduct a vocational assessment with you in order to identify your transferable skills and your new job goals. Agency personnel can also provide you with neuropsychological testing, which includes not only intellectual assessment but specific testing relating to memory, speed of information processing, and other cognitive concerns that may affect you as someone with MS. As reviewed in chapter 10, neuropsychological assessment is extremely helpful in enabling people to identify cognitive strengths and areas of weakness that need to be accommodated or worked around. As your job placement effort comes into focus, a state agency counselor may pay for other services for you, such as personal adjustment counseling, clothing for job interviews, support with transportation or gas funding, and so forth.

Often, the most helpful aid a state vocational rehabilitation counselor can provide is direct job placement assistance if you need it. This could include hiring a community placement specialist to work with you as someone seeking a full- or part-time job. In some instances, a rehabilitation consultant can be hired to establish a home-based position or assist you with a self-employment plan. You may or may not need direct representation in getting a job, but many others do need some representation from a rehabilitation agency. This may be due to the specific job being sought or to specific accommodation needs. In other instances, because of cognitive concerns, some job coaching or paid coworker mentoring may be needed, so that you can learn critical job skills to keep a job. State vocational rehabilitation (VR) may also pay part of your salary during a period of on-the-job training (OJT) with an employer. If you have no transferable skills, this last item may be your fastest route to new employment and financial stability.

Community Job Tryout: Department of Labor (DOL) Waiver

If it is unknown whether you can continue to work at your job or work effectively in relation to a new job goal, a community-based assessment or work trial period can be extremely beneficial. Under the 1993 Department of Labor (DOL) waiver (see appendix B), an individual with disability has a total of 215 hours to try out a nonpaid job for purposes of vocational exploration, establishing task proficiency, and training or skill-building.

The state vocational rehabilitation counselor often will pay a community rehabilitation provider to establish a community-based assessment (CBA) using this DOL waiver. If you are someone with MS, and you are experiencing fatigue, pain, new learning challenges, or other problems, and you need to try out some type of cognitive or physical accommodation, using these 215 hours can be quite helpful. You may need to present the DOL waiver to your state rehabilitation counselor (see appendix B) because many counselors are unfamiliar with it. Unfortunately, most people in personnel or human resources departments are also unfamiliar with this "tryout approach." The 215 hours, of course, do not need to be used completely; some individuals try out for only a few days or weeks to get the information they need.

If you are on medication and recovering either from initial symptoms or an exacerbation of MS, you may want to try out a job on the unpaid basis (e.g., beginning a few

> **TIP:** Copy appendix B and have it with you to consult, if necessary, while you are interviewing. It can be your ticket to getting back to work!

hours a day with gradual increases) in order to establish the accommodations that will work for you, including the length of your workday. In other cases, it may be more important to establish what you would enjoy doing in a certain type of job, and gain some experience in that activity. Some people can determine their comfort level and work capacity only by utilizing this tryout mechanism (e.g., twenty-five hours a week or a staggered three-day workweek).

Labor and Industry Insurance Costs

The Labor and Industry (L&I) insurance costs are typically paid by the state vocational rehabilitation agency or by the specific rehabilitation provider that has set up the tryout for you and is monitoring your progress. **Note:** Although the 215 hours granted to you adds up to less than six weeks when employed full-time, working only a few hours a day and graduating upwards can involve several months. This may be critical information for you as you mount a full-blown effort at working, versus the effort to move toward disability insurance or Social Security Disability Income (SSDI). Finally, you might decide to pursue SSDI, but work part-time and earn less than Substantial Gainful Activity (SGA), which is currently set by the Social Security Administration at about $830 monthly (periodically adjusted upward).

FINDING A JOB ON YOUR OWN

You might be ineligible for state vocational rehabilitation services due to your personal financial status and your savings or the earnings of your spouse or significant other. You may then have to seek a new full- or part-time job on your own. If you are certain of a job goal based on your education and prior work experience, you can target your efforts and use your state's WorkSource offices (see the upcoming section WorkSource: The State Employment Agency), Web site searches, and so forth.

If your goal is not clear to you, often vocational counseling can be obtained from an area community or state college on a nonpaid or paid basis. Also, you can choose to hire a private rehabilitation counselor or counseling psychologist. The National Multiple Sclerosis Society Web site can be very helpful for dealing with employment decisions and issues. The national Epilepsy Foundation Web site's, "Career Support Center" workstation linked to "Programs" on the home page is ideally linked to job search Web sites for those with and without a disability. It is a splendid resource.

Targeting Your Job Goal

Rumrill (1996, 81) and others have suggested that to be successful in your job search, you must identify the following: (a) specific job options, (b) geographical area(s) of focus, (c) the work values that are important to you, and (d) a series of potential contacts who can aid you in securing positions in this area(s).

In some instances, it will be difficult to identify job options immediately and you will need to consider using vocational interest inventories, such as the Strong Interest Inventory, the Career Assessment Inventory, or a state occupational information system inventory (as available on the Internet), in order to develop new goals. Counselors at community colleges, universities, and state employment offices can help you to "tweak" and refine your goals for your particular residential area. These counselors are often "low-cost" or "free" when compared to the fees charged by private counselors or psychologists.

Career development classes, taken through college or community college extension departments, can be helpful, although they may be less than optimal. As soon as your goals have been identified, certain types of short-term training can be invaluable to secure positions such as medical coder, medical billing specialist, security system installer, pest-control technician, and so forth. Other types of training are more long-term and the question for each individual is "How much time can be devoted to retraining, given your age and financial needs?"

Getting Through an Employer's Door

The focus of your job search is securing interviews, not simply mailing or e-mailing your résumés." Note that informational interviews are easier to schedule than actual job interviews, but they are very important in this job-seeking process and are invaluable for developing a contact base and for networking. Informational interviews still can require very targeted and consistent efforts from you.

Checklist 10: Getting Informational Interviews

The steps below, in checklist format, describe a systematic procedure for you to get some informational interviews (e.g., twenty-eight well-targeted mailings can result in five to eight informational interviews). Once the informational interview has been secured, your job will be to maximize the value of these interviews.

1. Have I identified my job goal? _____

2. Is my résumé established and refined (with critiques) from professional/significant others? _____

3. Have I a cover letter that asks for an informational interview in relation to a specific type of job? _____

4. Have I developed my "mass" mailing list to include specific contacts (names) from targeted areas of Chamber of Commerce directories, telephone yellow pages, business associations, unions, and other relevant groups? _____

5. Did I conduct my mass mailing and develop a tracking book? _____

6. All my targeted individuals are to be called within ten days from mailing the informational interview requests. If informational interview request is denied or the interview is unsuccessful relative to job procurement, did I ask interviewer for the names of other potential contacts? _____

   (Note: In each informational interview, employers can be informed about the incentives for hiring a qualified worker with a disability, e.g., tax credits, on-the-job training funding from state vocational rehabilitation office, federal tax deductions and credits for worksite accommodations, and any other incentives for employers to hire disabled workers. See appendix C.)

7. All informational interviewers and contacts identified through them are followed up every two weeks. _____

If no progress is made after a period of months, establish a new job goal and return to step 1 above to redo the entire process. Note that it is important to maintain tracking forms to follow up on your mass mailing. You can use the following example in worksheet 16 as a model for your tracking form.

WORKSHEET 16: MASS MAILING TRACKING FORM						
Contacts	Company Address	Phone	Called for Interview Y/N	Interview Date	Follow-ups	Other Information
1.						
2.						
3.						
4.						
5.						
6.						
7.						
8.						
9.						
10.						

There are many resources to help you develop your cover letter and refine your résumé. See Ryan's *Job Search Handbook for People with Disabilities* (2000). The informational interview will give you an opportunity to establish rapport with someone in your desired field, update your job-market information, get advice on your job search, obtain referrals, and so forth. When calling for the interview, make sure the employer knows that you are simply seeking information and do not want to take more than twenty minutes of his or her time. Be prepared for the following:

■ Discuss your background and goals for three to four minutes.

■ Describe five or more of your special skills and personal qualities as a part of this three-to-four minute presentation.

■ Be prepared to ask the employer questions about the company's job(s) of interest to you and about the company itself. Draw out the employer by your interest in (and knowledge of) the company.

- If your background is inadequate or barriers are presented, seek feedback for overcoming them. Also, ask feedback about your résumé.

GENERAL EMPLOYMENT RESOURCES

A number of state, federal, and local resources are described in this chapter. Many of them can be linked to your locale through the Epilepsy Foundation Web site Career Support Center link as mentioned previously.

WorkSource: The State Employment Agency

WorkSource state employment agencies are located throughout each state. These centers offer employers all the information, technology, and personal services that are available for finding and hiring employees. You can post your résumé in the state WorkSource databank for potential matching to an employer's needs within your community. Career counseling is available, but the quality can vary both within and across states.

You, however, have access to the Internet and to public and private job search engines. If you were laid off or terminated from a position, you can receive your unemployment insurance payments (if eligible) through these centers as long as you maintain active job seeking. You may have access to short-term retraining funds and almost all WorkSource sites conduct classes on job search and job maintenance.

Several partnering agencies, such as state vocational rehabilitation, emergency retraining programs, and so on, often can be found at these sites. The concept behind WorkSource is to house or link all available employment resources within the one site. Contact with a disability specialist, veteran's specialist, or other advocate (as appropriate) at the site can turn out to be invaluable to you.

National Multiple Sclerosis Society Affiliates and Other MS Associations

Although most MS affiliates or associations don't have employment programs, a few do have them. Or you may be referred to a knowledgeable state vocational rehabilitation agency provider or other well-informed vocational rehabilitation service providers. Staff at these associations are also informed about SSDI issues, application procedures and strategies, discrimination issues, and so on, and they can be helpful on a number of employment-related matters.

Kent State University Employment Assistance Service, Akron, Ohio

The above-named service, under the direction of Dr. Phil Rumrill, actually can provide you with MS-specific job accommodation recommendations at no cost if your local MS association has a subscription with them. Unfortunately, to date, only the following affiliates have subscribed to this service for their clients: Greater Illinois (Chicago); Georgia; Channel Islands (Santa Barbara, California); Greater Connecticut (Hartford to New York suburbs); Northeast Ohio (including Columbus); Ohio Valley (Cincinnati); and Mid-South (most of Tennessee and part of North Carolina). Hopefully, this service soon will expand to your area.

The Ticket to Work Program

The Social Security Administration developed the national Ticket to Work program in which an individual on a Social Security subsidy can be assigned a voucher that can be utilized by any certified employment network (EN) within a state in order to provide that person with job-placement assistance. These employment networks can be diverse: vocational and social services agencies, or businesses within your community, and all state vocational rehabilitation agencies will be ENs. These networks get paid only when you (as a person with Social Security support) secure a job that is substantial gainful activity (SGA) and you terminate your Social Security Disability Income (SSDI) or your Supplemental Security Income (SSI). If the position does not work out, you may get back onto SSDI or SSI automatically, with any accompanying medical coverage. Your "employability" will then be reevaluated while the Social Security subsidy and Medicaid coverage are provided.

The Ticket to Work program was also developed with the assumption that an individual might be using a state's buy-in mechanism relative to Medicaid if the employer does not provide health insurance. Given national economic constraints, this option may not always be available and you may need to evaluate your medical needs very carefully before dropping the support provided through Medicaid. Individuals seeking only part-time work (below $830 per month for SSDI) and wishing to maintain their SSDI or SSI support will not qualify for the Ticket to Work voucher. As of 2004, the Ticket to Work system was implemented in every state, but the program was poorly thought-out and it now has lost the confidence of Social Security administrators and may be reformatted as this book goes to press.

Church and Religious Groups

Many church and religious groups have made efforts to provide employment assistance for their parishioners and friends due to today's high unemployment levels. This can involve the establishment of a job bank, which is available to community members outside of the religious group. In many cases, this can involve support of a job search or a networking group at the facility. Your church or synagogue, therefore, should not be overlooked as a potential source of employment referrals. Many people list their desired job in the church or synagogue weekly newsletter, which is often distributed at religious services. Faith-based communities frequently want to take care of their own and may reach out to you.

Professional Trade Organizations

Some associations (e.g., medical associations) have their own employment office reflecting the diverse employment needs of their members. In other instances, union and other trade associations have representatives who may know about apprentice and other training access routes for those seeking work in a specific field.

Temporary Jobs

Although you may have a specific job goal in mind, it can be beneficial to work one to two days per week (or more) at a temporary job. This would be not only for your cash flow, but also to increase your job-related contacts within your community. Temporary work is also helpful in alleviating depression and anxiety. Today, many temporary employment agencies provide a range of both skilled and unskilled employees to employers. Some companies will hire permanently only from the temporary pool of workers currently working for them. (This is known as "temp to perm" hiring.) Basically, these companies use the temporary help option as a screening mechanism for hiring quality permanent employees. Temporary agencies are a burgeoning access point to viable jobs in our economy.

College/Training Facility Employment Offices and Former Teachers

Most colleges or training facilities allow their graduates to return to their job-placement offices despite the fact that they may be years away from graduation. This is a resource that is not to be overlooked. In some cases, individuals return to former teachers (some of whom assisted them in securing a first job) for leads and additional contacts. Contacts made through your prior training facility and your teachers may be very important and should be contacted regularly. Some teachers will refer you to successful alumni who will then make that extra effort for you as a fellow or sister alumnus.

Chambers of Commerce

Most Chambers of Commerce have a monthly (low- or no-cost) social gathering at which it can be reasonably easy to meet employers from your community. Don't miss them. Bring your résumé, your best social small talk, and your clearly prepared job goal conversation. Typically, Chamber of Commerce directories are categorized by different types of businesses, provide contact personnel, and are free or inexpensive from the organization. This can be a great resource for getting those informational interviews close to home. A local Chamber of Commerce may also provide access to a job close to home.

Fraternal and Charitable Organizations

Fraternal and charitable organizations such as Rotary, Elks, Shriners, or Kiwanis draw their membership from diverse community businesses. Try attending a meeting as a guest of a member and when you are introduced, be prepared to discuss your job goal succinctly. Every Rotary club in the world has a Vocational Services committee. Try to contact this committee's chairperson to make your job needs known. Such organizational officers are generally receptive and may make the extra effort to make member contacts for you.

Conclusion

Hopefully, this chapter has provided you with a starting point for planning your job maintenance strategy or your job search efforts. Efforts were made to provide you with a range of available community resources. The descriptions provided are not exhaustive. Other resources can be identified through your local chapter of the National Multiple Sclerosis Society. You are limited only by your own creativity in these areas. Take breaks when your job search becomes exhausting, but stay the course because ultimately it can be very rewarding (in multiple ways) to be a member of the workforce.

CHAPTER 8

Disclosure to Employer and Using Job Accommodations

Kurt L. Johnson, Ph.D., C.R.C.

WHY DO WE WORK?

All of us work for many reasons. Certainly, bringing home income is critical, as is the security of having employer-paid health insurance. Perhaps less obvious is the sense of purpose that comes with working. Work can be an important part of your identity. In the workplace, you have the opportunity to demonstrate your skills and to experience recognition for your competence and to achieve success. Finally, your workplace provides you with opportunities for positive social interactions. As you most likely know, when you have multiple sclerosis (MS), issues around work may become complicated.

When you have MS, working can have costs as well as benefits. For example, work can be very tiring. You can get so tired during the workday that when you get home from work, you have no energy left for leisure or even for necessary activities such as shopping. Some people living with MS find that they must choose between working and having a good quality of life after work.

Also, work can be stressful, particularly if you are experiencing cognitive changes, fatigue, or pain. When you have cognitive changes such as difficulty with memory and multitasking, it takes energy and focus to think effectively and efficiently. You may have to become more vigilant to make sure that you say what you want to say. For some, this extra effort leads to greater fatigue, which promotes further difficulty in thinking. When you experience a combination of some of these factors, interactions with your coworkers and supervisors may become quite stressful.

On the other hand, being unemployed, not having health insurance, and being home alone also can be very stressful. As one person in our qualitative research study noted,

I don't think about being tired when I'm at work—my mind is too busy to think about my legs hurting. That's the best reason why people should work. You forget about the MS. If I am home, I get really depressed.

So, you have to balance the costs and the benefits you experience by working and then you will be in a better position to make a decision about employment that works for you and your family.

BARRIERS TO WORKING

So let's assume that you've decided either to continue working or to reenter the workplace. What are the barriers that you may encounter? And what kind of strategies can you use to address these barriers? First of all, let's not underestimate how significant these barriers may be. Given their educational level and age, people with MS are unemployed at a much higher rate than would be expected (Law and Noyes 2005). Since about 70 percent of those with MS are women, and they are usually diagnosed in their twenties (Kurtzke 2005), some of this unemployment may be due to the fact that some women may have been out of the labor market during their childbearing years. However, from the research, it looks as though people with MS leave the labor market prematurely (Fraser, McMahon, and Danczyk-Hawley 2003). Moreover, in surveys of people with MS, many who are unemployed say they wish they could have a job, and those who continue to work place a high value on their employment (LaRocca and Hall 1990; LaRocca et al. 1985). So we will begin by looking at employment barriers that are related to having MS, and later we will look at barriers to employment that are related to society or to the work environment.

Fatigue

Fatigue can come in many different forms. Sometimes, you may wake up in the morning and be so dead tired that you can't even begin to think about going to work; that kind of fatigue can continue for several days. Often, this kind of fatigue is associated with an exacerbation of MS. So, if you experience this kind of fatigue periodically, when you address accommodations for fatigue in your workplace, it will be important for your physician to document that this is not just about being tired. Significant fatigue associated with your MS is a legitimate reason for you to miss work. When you are this tired, most likely it isn't even feasible for you to try to work from home until your energy picks up again.

More frequently, though, you may find that you experience more fatigue as your workday progresses. For this kind of fatigue, it will be helpful if you can figure out a pattern. For example, if you know that you usually have more energy in the morning, you may be able to schedule important activities earlier in the day. Also, you might notice that you get really tired around lunchtime, in which case, as a reasonable accommodation, you might request that you be allowed to combine your lunch break with your afternoon break so you can take a nap. Some clients in our employment programs set a timer and nap in their car, or they use a cot or floor mat for rest, or they actually go home for a couple of hours of sleep, returning for the late afternoon shift (e.g., 3:30–6:30 P.M.). Other clients refresh themselves with a timed fifteen-minute nap in the afternoon.

Some people have had great success learning and using relaxation techniques, such as progressive muscle relaxation, meditation, or meditative prayer. They find that deep relaxation for ten or fifteen minutes, two or three times during the day "recharges their batteries." And, as one individual explained, "MS fatigue is different. When those of us with MS use the word 'fatigue,' you might think 'tired,' but it's different. Our reserves are depleted and they don't refill; you can't refill them." Finally, some medications, such as amantadine or provigil, have proved effective for some people with MS in combating fatigue. You can discuss their use with your physician.

Cognitive Changes

Cognitive changes in the workplace can be very tough and may require strategic thinking to accommodate. Cognitive changes might include difficulties with memory, paying attention to tasks, and problem solving (particularly under pressure). There also may be problems with thinking more slowly, having difficulty finding words, or having difficulty with multitasking. As one person described it, "There are cognitive problems. I don't think as clearly as I used to. That doesn't mean I can't do my job, but it is more of a struggle."

Managing fatigue and heat sensitivity will be important because you may have more difficulty with cognitive tasks when you are too hot or more tired. If you can, schedule your more demanding activities for morning hours. One woman with MS goes to work two hours before her coworkers arrive so she can concentrate on complex financial tasks, without the distractions of coworkers' voices and telephones ringing, and so forth. She schedules less demanding tasks for afternoons when she is less efficient cognitively. Additionally, she tries to schedule her phone calls for an hour in the early afternoon so she can focus on one function at a time. When she gets home, she routinely takes a nap, so by the time her husband gets home from his job, she is rested enough to enjoy some quality time with him.

Three Rules to Help with Cognitive Changes

The primary rule in accommodating your cognitive changes is routine, routine, routine! The idea behind insisting on routines to follow is that the more activities that are predictable, routine, simple, and automatic, the more physical or cognitive energy you will have available to apply to higher-level activities.

This primary rule begins with what may seem simple, but for many of us is difficult: unclutter your work space. Removing distractions by making sure that unnecessary papers and objects are filed away (or discarded) will help you to work much more efficiently. Also, it can be very helpful to have a daily reminder system with a to-do list and a good filing system so that you can schedule time to remember what's the next item on your work list.

Let's look at an example of the cluttered desk. Shown below are two photos of a "before and after" intervention that was done for a woman having difficulties attending to her tasks at her workstation. Although this was a relatively simple intervention, the difference it makes in her ability to get her job done is obvious.

The second rule might be repetition, repetition, repetition! When you find it more difficult to learn new material, or to understand complex material, repetition may help. One woman with MS said that when she was younger, she would quickly scan complex reports before meetings with clients and retain enough information to hold her own. Now that she has some cognitive problems, she reads the reports the evening before her meeting, highlights relevant sections with a highlighting pen, and then scans the highlights the next day just before the meeting. This takes her about twice as long, but it allows her to be well prepared and effective during her client meetings. Other people with MS tape-record highlighted material for themselves and review the audiotape several times before key meetings.

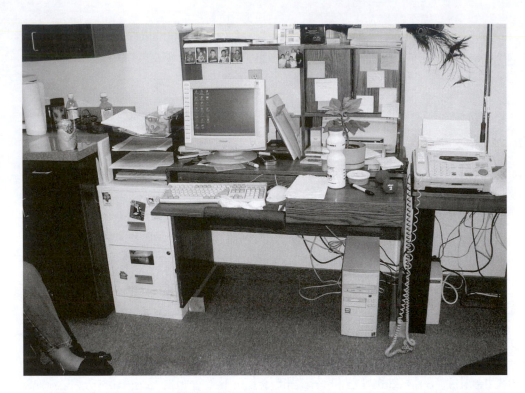

Figure 8.1: This "before" photo shows the cluttered work space of a woman with MS. She asked for assistance because it was difficult for her to focus on her work.

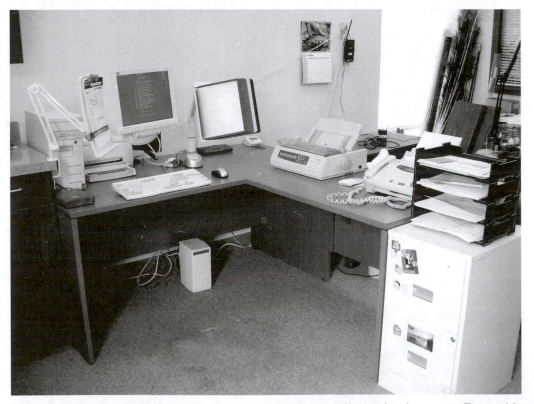

Figure 8.2: In this "after" photo, the work space has been redesigned to be more efficient. Notice that all materials are organized and the clutter is gone. A flat-panel computer monitor has replaced the old monitor, freeing up desk space. A new desk was provided that allows her to easily move from activity to activity in her wheelchair.

The third rule might be organize, organize, organize! Think about the scope and flow of your work. What kinds of things do you need to remember? What kind of strategy will work best for you personally? For some people a daily planner is just the ticket. You can use it as your memory book. Not only can you write down all your appointments, you also can take notes in the Notes section, maintain a to-do list, and have references to important notes or tasks in your calendar. You can find different organizing systems at most office or business supply stores. Speech and language pathologists knowledgeable about memory can also help design customized tools and strategies.

Electronic Devices

What about electronic devices? Anything that you do with a daily planner, you can certainly do with a personal digital assistant (PDA) running either the Palm OS® or the Pocket PC®. The advantages of these systems are that they have alarms that can be set to remind you to check them and they have multilayered, sophisticated organizing systems such as Microsoft Outlook®. The disadvantage of PDAs is that it may be difficult to learn to use them if you are not comfortable with the technology. Also, you must make sure the battery is charged and data are backed up.

Some people with MS set up their desktop computers to help them work more efficiently. For example, using Microsoft Outlook®, they have set up their e-mail so that it sorts messages into logical boxes, making it easier to see what needs to be attended to quickly. One woman showed me how she had used color coding. For the same reasons that were discussed regarding your work space, you should make sure that the desktop on your computer is organized and uncluttered.

Many people with MS have told the author that they use e-mail as a memory aid. They e-mail messages to themselves so they can remember to update their calendars and their to-do lists. You can also use a text pager or a cell phone as a memory aid. Your computer can send text messages from the schedule in Outlook to your cell phone or to your text pager, reminding you of important activities. A low-tech version is used simply to call your home or cell telephone message service and leave yourself reminders.

Depression

As described in chapter 5, depression is common among people with MS. And, as you can imagine, because of the relationship between depression, fatigue, and pain, depression can be quite a barrier to employment. Therefore, if you have any concerns about depression, I recommend that you review chapter 5 and seek treatment from someone knowledgeable about both depression and MS.

Pain

In the research literature, between 44 to 80 percent of those with MS report that they have pain (Ehde, Osborne, and Jensen 2005). Because pain can be intrusive and increase fatigue, it will be important to minimize the impact of pain at work, and in your life in general. This may require medical intervention and, perhaps, managing your activity patterns. Obviously, the medical intervention route requires a trip to your healthcare provider and a description of the pain that you feel. Managing your activity patterns may include taking strategic breaks at work, ensuring that you are as rested as you can be, and taking time-outs so you can use cognitive strategies to help disrupt your pain.

Heat Sensitivity

Approximately 80 percent of people with MS report some kind of heat sensitivity (Halper 2005). They say that mostly they don't do as well when they are too warm as they do when they are cool. Occasionally, some people with MS are sensitive to cold. In the workplace, a request that you be provided with control over the temperature in your work area would be a very reasonable accommodation. In warmer climates or seasons, limiting your trips outdoors during the hotter part of the day is sensible. Air-conditioning for your car during commutes can be critical.

It also may be beneficial in general to carry a thermos of iced water with you in warm weather. In some cases, a simple, portable air-conditioner in the work area is sufficient. If you are extremely sensitive to heat, a cooling jacket or a heat-extraction system may really boost your tolerance for work. Cooling jackets are unobtrusive garments worn by people with MS, they provide a personal cooling system. Your physician will be able to review your options. Heat-extraction systems are worn on the body as vests or jackets and are either pre-cooled or attached to portable devices that cool continuously.

Mobility

You may be one of those with MS who experience difficulty with mobility. Some people find that they tire very quickly when walking. Others are unsteady, have difficulty walking, and some are unable to walk. To address limitations in mobility, you can use basic mobility aids such as canes, walkers, or wheelchairs. Difficulty with mobility can have an impact on work from many different perspectives. Getting to and from work may take more time and effort. Traveling distances while at your work site may take more energy and time. Some jobs require that employees travel off the worksite, or even out of town, and mobility limitations can pose significant challenges in this area.

Finally, nonwork activities can come into play. If walking is tiring or difficult, activities such as shopping for food may take much more energy and planning, depleting energy stores for the next workday. If you find this to be true, you may want to conserve your energy by shopping online or by using the phone for groceries and other items, and having them delivered to your home. Or a friend or volunteer might pick up your packages for you. Making quarterly bulk purchases for staples and frozen food items at low-cost grocery outlets and warehouses can save you time and money.

For people who tire easily when walking, there are a couple of potential accommodations that may help. First, it may be possible to move your office or desk to reduce the walking distance to the restroom, cafeteria, or parking area. One woman told me she was able to reduce her walking by 50 percent simply by switching offices with a coworker. Mobility aids, such as modified walkers with seats, can help you feel more stable and give you a place

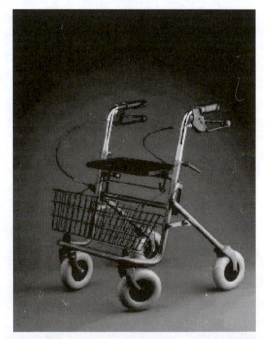

Figure 8.3: This is an example of a modified walker with a seat for resting. Notice that it has hand brakes for additional stability and a basket for carrying objects. You can see how you could sit and rest on this while waiting for a bus, and then fold it up to board the bus.

Figure 8.4: This is an example of a power scooter. These are light enough that many people can disassemble them independently to place them in the trunk of their car for transport.

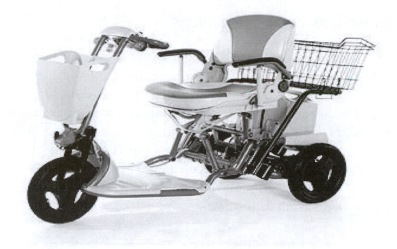

Figure 8.5: This power wheelchair is similar to the one used by the woman described below. These chairs are expensive, beginning at around $6,000 and they must be transported by a van with a lift or ramp. Options for these types of equipment can be reviewed with your physician, occupational therapist, your local multiple sclerosis organizations, or through the Job Accommodation Network (JAN) on the Internet.

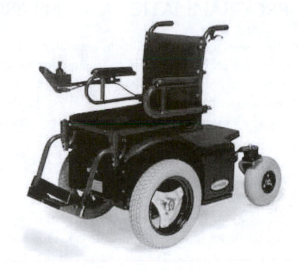

to sit and rest periodically. The range of options includes the use of various power mobility aids, including scooters and power wheelchairs. These can be used not only at work but in all environments.

One woman told me that she was becoming very fatigued from the walking she had to do while at work. She applied for services with the state Department of Vocational Rehabilitation for assistance in maintaining her employment. They provided her with an evaluation of her mobility needs at work and, as a result, purchased a power wheelchair for her to use.

She decided to use the power wheelchair only at work because it would have been very expensive for her to buy a van to transport the chair, and it was not convenient for her to use public transportation in the power wheelchair. Also, her apartment was small and would not have accommodated a wheelchair easily. Her employer moved her to a larger office, and the building owner built a locking cabinet in the parking garage where she can leave her wheelchair when she isn't at work.

She said that this solution reduced her fatigue and pain significantly, and she discovered that she now can join her colleagues when they lunch at restaurants in the neighborhood. The wheelchair increased her ability to engage with others both in her occupation and in her social life.

Bladder and Bowel Difficulties

Bladder dysfunction is one of the top five most prominent symptoms affecting the quality of life for people with MS (Rothwell et al. 1997). Nevertheless, if you have experienced persistent bowel and bladder difficulties, understandably you find these very distressing, even imprisoning. The causes of bladder and bowel problems vary with disease function, as do interventions which can range from managing fluid intake and caution with diet, to use of a condom, intermittent or indwelling catheters, medications, or, occasionally, surgery. If you are having bladder or bowel problems, consult your healthcare provider right away and, if necessary, ask for a referral to a specialist such as a urologist familiar with neurological disability who can help you devise a management strategy that will limit the interference at work and in your community.

SOCIAL, PROGRAMMATIC, AND ENVIRONMENTAL BARRIERS

It's clear from the research about disability in general, and MS in particular, that many of the barriers to employment are not related to the functional limitations you can experience as someone with MS; rather they are related to social attitudes, policy issues like healthcare insurance benefits, and environmental variables such as temperature and curb cuts. These barriers can be difficult to detect and can be powerfully disabling, so it is important that you consider them carefully.

Social Barriers

When you encounter problems related to MS at work, it's natural that your family and healthcare provider may suggest that you should quit your job. You, however, may very well continue working with the appropriate accommodations. The economic and social consequences of unemployment may be more stressful than working. So, it's important to recognize that the suggestions you receive are just that—suggestions. They reflect the attitudes of those around you, without consideration of the complex issues you are facing. Be especially cautious about making decisions about employment *during* an exacerbation. First, let matters stabilize, and then take your time to make the decision that will be best for you. Consider the advice you're getting from those around you, but also think about using the planning process we describe below to make sure you take into consideration all of your areas of concern.

Assuming the people in your workplace know you have MS (there will be more about disclosure later in this chapter), your employer or coworkers may over- or underestimate the degree of your level of disability. They may believe that because you have difficulty speaking clearly or walking steadily when you are fatigued, that you are cognitively impaired. What's more, they may not share that perception with you and then make decisions about the tasks that are assigned to you or the promotions you receive based on their incorrect perceptions. These attitudes and beliefs can result in discrimination and have a negative impact on your work. As one woman with MS put it, "I think basically you get stereotyped and they see you as your ailment and they don't see you for yourself."

There are a variety of ways to confront attitudinal barriers. You may choose not to disclose that you have MS in the workplace. You may try educating your coworkers or employers during a relaxed period in the workday (e.g., at a break or at lunchtime). Since the passage of the Americans with Disabilities Act (ADA) of 1990, discrimination in employment against people with disabilities (which affect one or more major life areas) who can perform the essential functions of the job (with or without accommodation) is illegal. If you cannot recommend a specific accommodation for yourself, under ADA the company has a responsibility to seek technical consultation (e.g., an occupational therapist or assistive technologist for physical issues and a neuropsychologist or speech and language pathologist for cognitive concerns).

Programmatic Barriers

Programmatic barriers to employment can be formidable. You may feel that you can't change jobs because that would require you to change your healthcare insurance, and a new policy would exclude MS treatment as a preexisting condition (see chapter 9 for full discussion of this issue). Also, you may feel that you must quit work because you need governmental healthcare coverage, such as Medicare or Medicaid, to pay for your medical care and medications. Perhaps you've discovered that the special medications you take for your MS are covered under your major medical coverage rather than your prescription drug coverage, thus requiring a big outlay of cash from you every month. The lack of universal health care coverage in the U.S., and the absence of consistency in employer-funded healthcare coverage plans can put those who have MS into very difficult positions with respect to employment.

Furthermore, there are other kinds of programmatic issues you may have to face. For example, is there a good public transportation system in your area? If so, is it fully accessible to people with disabilities? Does the local governmental office of civil rights consider disability issues to be a priority? Are services available from the state Department of Vocational Rehabilitation? Is there an interdisciplinary team associated with your healthcare provider who can help you identify appropriate accommodations? If not, you may want to seek a consultation through a more comprehensive MS center.

Environmental Barriers

Finally, let's consider environmental barriers. Climate can be a big environmental barrier for people with heat sensitivity. Would you function better in Miami, Florida, or Seattle, Washington, in the summer? Climate can also be a big barrier for people who have difficulty with mobility. Would you rather navigate the winter snow in Buffalo, New York, or the rain of Eugene, Oregon? And what about terrain? Would you rather climb (on foot or with your mobility device) the hills of San Francisco or the level streets with bike lanes in Davis, California? And what about elevators and curb cuts? Can you travel from where you live to work and to key points in your community without experiencing obstructions?

Unfortunately, despite the legal requirements of the Americans with Disabilities Act, some communities remain relatively inaccessible to people with disabilities. One of our clients recently sold a home in Seattle to winter in Florida and live with family in a Long Island beach town in the summer, both for the climate and support needs. Moving to a more disability-friendly or accessible community might be a realistic option for your consideration.

DEVELOPING YOUR PERSONAL ACCOMMODATION PLAN

Now, let's put this all together and discuss your personal accommodation plan. After reviewing the barriers and potential solutions described in this chapter, turn to the back of this book, and take some time to carefully review the Work Experience Survey (Roessler and Gottcent 1994) in appendix A. You will then be in a better position to make a few important decisions: Is it in your best interests to continue working (or get a job)? Should you disclose to your employer that you have MS? What kinds of accommodations would be useful to you at work and who should pay for them?

Dr. Roessler recommends that sections II–V of the Work Experience Survey (see appendix A) can be used, more easily, to better clarify your barriers to employment, potential solutions, and the "who" and "how" of each solution. You can also take the results of your efforts and seek assistance from a rehabilitation counselor, a speech and language pathologist (familiar with neurological and cognitive rehabilitation), a rehabilitation counselor or neuropsychologist, an assistive technology specialist, or other professional recommended by your healthcare provider, state vocational rehabilitation agency, or local MS organization.

There are also a number of resources available on the Web. For example, you can learn more about your legal rights from the Department of Justice Web site (see Resources). Information about how to accommodate your job barriers can be found at the Job Accommodation Network (JAN) and information about useful equipment or assistive technology can be found at ABLEDATA (see Resources section at the end of the book). Using JAN as an example, you pose your barrier and accommodation question on the Web site and, usually, you will receive a recommendation for accommodation by e-mail within a day. Options can include the manner in which certain companies make accommodations, the offerings of the manufacturers of assistive technologies or adaptive software, and even journal articles comparing the benefits of different accommodation strategies. Having worked through this process, you will then be better prepared to discuss your needs with your current or prospective employer.

It's important to think through how the potential accommodation costs will be covered: By your employer? By you? By a state vocational rehabilitation agency? By some combination? Fortunately, most accommodations are inexpensive, costing less than $500. Often, the accommodation needed is simply a procedural change (e.g., modifying your work schedule versus physical modification to the workstation itself).

DISCLOSING TO YOUR EMPLOYER

So, now let's presume you have decided to keep working or to get a job, and that accommodations would be useful on the job. Should you tell your employer that you have MS? For some people, it may be difficult not to disclose since others can see they have a disability of some kind because they use a wheelchair, have difficulty with speech, and so on. But for others, MS may be an "invisible" disability, and the decision to disclose is up to the individual.

You may choose not to specifically reference multiple sclerosis, but simply disclose that you have a disability that affects you in certain ways and requires certain accommodation. This is your call and you may want to discuss this with your physician, spouse, and significant others.

On the other hand, disclosing to the employer is necessary to establish your legal rights. And, from a practical perspective, it may be difficult to negotiate even small accommodations, such as modified breaks to allow brief naps, without explaining why they are needed.

Usually, disclosure to an employer is appropriate only when you are making a request for a "reasonable accommodation." Under the ADA, and many state laws, if you are a "qualified individual with a disability" (your MS affects "one or more major life areas"), and you can perform the "essential functions of your job" (that would be the functions that are clearly central to your job), "with or without accommodation," and your employer is a "covered entity" (under federal law, the company is a "covered entity" if your employer has twenty-five or more employees; and under some state laws, the company is a covered entity if your employer has as few as eight employees), your employer is required to pay for "reasonable accommodations" necessary for you to do your job, and cannot discriminate against you because of your disability. "Reasonable" is not defined, but is based on administrative regulations and case law. What is reasonable depends on the size of the employer, the amount of revenue, and other factors. The "reasonable accommodation" cannot impose an "undue hardship" on the employer. Unfortunately, if you have MS and are in remission or have fewer symptoms than most people with MS, you may not be covered under ADA, although you may be covered under state law.

So, to whom do you make your request for accommodation? With larger employers, that request is usually made to the Human Resources department. Some larger companies will have a Disability Services Unit with vocational rehabilitation counselors on the staff. Under the law, you are not required to disclose that you have MS, but you must state that you have a disability, and you must state the functional limitations you want to address with the accommodations. Your employer has the right to request verification of your functional limitations from your physician, but you have the right to ask your physician to document the limitations but *not to include the diagnosis*.

For example, you could ask your physician to verify that you have significant fatigue that is unpredictable and you need flexibility in your schedule to accommodate your fatigue; and that with that accommodation, you can do your job, but if you choose not to mention MS, you don't have to. There are no right or wrong answers here. The decisions about whether to disclose and what to disclose are very personal. You may find that you feel more comfortable telling your supervisor and coworkers, or you may cherish your privacy. Again, you may decide to find your own accommodations. Of course, making different decisions will have different consequences.

Worksheet 17 below reviews your decision-making process. Note that if you decide not to work and to pursue Social Security Disability Income, medical retirement, and so forth, you may be able to do some part-time work (based on your capacity for work) that is not considered substantial gainful activity (SGA). This can be reviewed with a vocational rehabilitation counselor or Social Security representative. If you are considering some part-time work, you still will need to consider the disclosure issue. When going through the process, you will need separate sheets of paper for your observations in relation to decision-process points A, B, C, F, and G, H, and I. Information in relation to your limitations and solutions/accommodations can be developed by using the Work Experience Survey you will find in appendix A.

Conclusion

When you have MS, the decision about whether to work can be very complex. Psychological, social, and economic variables all come into play. When you have difficulty with some elements of work because of your MS, accommodations can be very helpful. Often accommodations are simple, inexpensive, and common sense (e.g., using a day planner). At other times, however, such as when you need to reduce your work-related travel or modify a restroom door, you may need to consider disclosing your MS, or at least your fundamental limitations, to your employer. You can then request that the employer pay for or assist with the accommodation, seek accommodation funds from a state vocational rehabilitation agency, or even pay for it yourself if it is not particularly costly and you wish to avoid bureaucratic red tape.

WORKSHEET 17:   SHOULD I DISCLOSE?

Disclosure Note: See worksheet 15 in chapter 7 for the disclosure script.

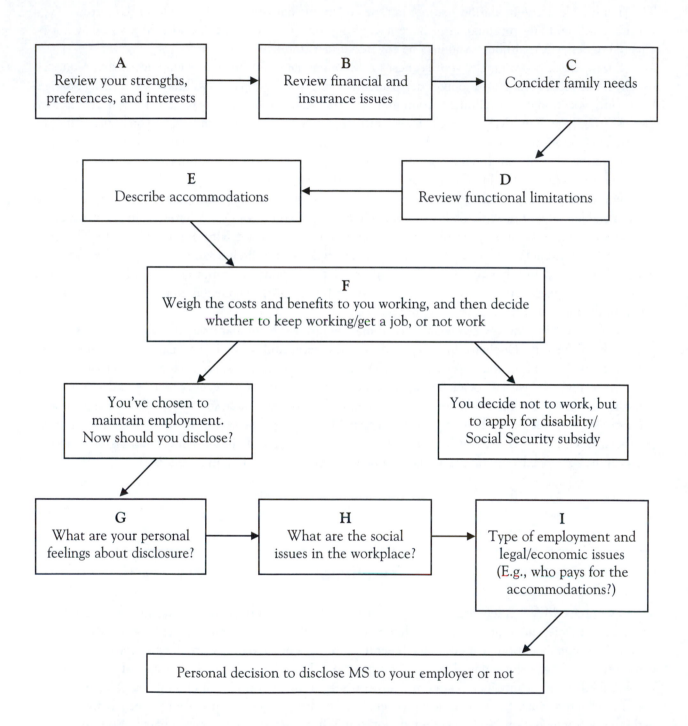

A
Review your strengths, preferences, and interests

B
Review financial and insurance issues

C
Concider family needs

D
Review functional limitations

E
Describe accommodations

F
Weigh the costs and benefits to you working, and then decide whether to keep working/get a job, or not work

You've chosen to maintain employment. Now should you disclose?

You decide not to work, but to apply for disability/ Social Security subsidy

G
What are your personal feelings about disclosure?

H
What are the social issues in the workplace?

I
Type of employment and legal/economic issues (E.g., who pays for the accommodations?)

Personal decision to disclose MS to your employer or not

CHAPTER 9

Dealing with Health Insurance and Financial Concerns

Robert T. Fraser, Ph.D., C.R.C. and Phillip R. Rumrill, Ph.D., C.R.C.

MS AND FINANCIAL CHALLENGES

As a person with multiple sclerosis (MS), you may be in early or mid-career at the time of your diagnosis. The initial decisions you make may include choices about continuing to work and maintaining your financial status. For most of you, this is obviously your best financial position. The following questions may seem obvious, but they are worth asking because their importance cannot be overstated. While you are working toward medical stabilization, have you used all of your available sick leave and vacation time? If you can work part-time or several days a week, have you spread out your vacation and sick days to the best of your ability? Perhaps some of your colleagues could donate some of their sick leave to you? Have you been creative with your Family and Medical Leave Act (FMLA) time? Note that some states offer disability leave that will pay a percentage of your salary while you are recuperating. Check with your local WorkSource office.

If the best efforts have been made medically and you've gone through the decision-making process described in chapter 8 and decided you are no longer able to stay at your job, then there still are a number of issues that must be handled. Your health insurance is, of course, of primary concern. Your company may have short- and long-term disability insurance, and this income stream must be considered. Then, the effort to secure Social Security benefits, that is, Social Security Disability Income (SSDI) for those with work experience or Supplemental Security Income (SSI) for those who were not working or have no extended work experience, must be considered.

Other issues relate to considering part-time work as a supplement to your SSDI subsidy and any work-related expenses that can reduce your income and, therefore, leave your Social Security benefits intact. Some of you must simply work toward establishing a "bottom line" of monthly financial assets and income stream versus mandatory debt. In sum, there are many issues to be considered in the financial planning area and dealing with these issues is the focus of this chapter.

KEEPING YOUR JOB

From a financial perspective, the initial focus for most of you will be on keeping your job. How much vacation and sick leave can you use? Does your company have short- and long-term disability insurance you can use? Could you let it be known through the employee network that you'd appreciate some donated sick leave time from colleagues? Can you meet the requirements for the Family and Medical Leave Act (FMLA) to tap into more time (albeit unpaid) in order to keep your job? The basic point here is that there are a number of options to be considered before you give up on a job that is meaningful and financially rewarding to you.

SHORT- AND LONG-TERM DISABILITY INSURANCE

The availability of support under disability insurance programs depends on the type of program to which your employer subscribes. Short-term disability programs usually provide coverage of 60 to 80 percent of salary for a period of time that can range from three months to two years. Long-term disability usually extends from short-term disability to retirement, but you will be required to apply for Social Security benefits, which when secured, are usually deducted from your benefits. For example, if your long-term disability insurance check is $2,000 per month and you obtain SSDI benefits of $1,100 per month, your long-term disability insurance payout will be reduced to $900 per month, bringing the total to the $2,000 per month that the insurer originally guaranteed to you.

HEALTH INSURANCE CONCERNS

If you do leave your job, obviously, health insurance coverage will be a major concern. There are a range of insurance options that may be available to you that are important to understand. They are discussed below.

The Consolidated Omnibus Budget Reconciliation Act (COBRA) of 1985

COBRA is a law requiring employers who offer group health insurance coverage to their employees to provide a continuation of their insurance after an employee's termination for a specified length of time. This Act usually covers the health plans of employers with twenty or more employees who have worked at least 50 percent of the workdays in the prior calendar year.

The insurance premiums of the terminated employee are paid at the company's group rate. COBRA benefits also extend to the spouse and dependents of the terminated employee. COBRA benefits are available for eighteen months after termination and may be extended for an additional eleven months in the event of disability.

You, your spouse, and your dependents may not be eligible for COBRA if you were not yet eligible for the group insurance program, were terminated due to gross misconduct, had declined group insurance coverage, or became eligible for Medicare. Spouses of former employees lose coverage if they divorce or separate or the former employee dies.

Health Insurance Portability and Accountability Act (HIPAA) of 1996

The emphasis of this Act was to provide access to group health plans for workers who wish to change jobs or are terminated. The coverage includes medical, dental, vision, prescription drugs, flexible spending accounts, and some employee/assistance plans. HIPAA limits exclusions for preexisting medical conditions that could force you to stay with the company that employs you. It also prohibits discrimination based on your disability and health status in the area of group insurance coverage.

Essentially, HIPAA establishes that if you were insured during the previous twelve months, you will have no waiting period under any new employer's group plan. You must, however, have been treated for your medical condition, in this case multiple sclerosis (MS), in the six-month period preceding new plan enrollment. You don't necessarily have to have seen your physician, but you would have had to be taking some medication or receiving treatment.

If you were not insured in the twelve months prior to applying for the new employer's insurance plan, your longest waiting period should be only twelve months. HIPAA also requires the issuance of a Certificate of Coverage for evidence of coverage of your preexisting condition to expedite coverage with your new insurer.

Individual Insurance Plans

If you have no new employer-insurance options and you've exhausted your COBRA benefits, a number of private medical insurance options may be available in your state. Acceptance is based on a point total from the new insurer's medical questionnaire. Monthly premium costs are based on your age and the deductible (e.g., $500, $1,000, etc.). The higher the deductible, the lower the premium. If you are rejected from assignment to one of these plans, you may then be eligible for state health insurance pools maintained by the majority of states for individuals considered to be high risk.

State Health Insurance for High Risk Individuals

If you are denied health insurance as a *high-risk* cost person, most states administer a high-risk health insurance pool. These programs provide insurance coverage and can provide it at a more reasonable rate than other insurers. Although eligibility can vary by state, many states use the federal standards of eligibility. Federal standards of eligibility include the following:

- You have exhausted your COBRA/state program benefits

- You had at least eighteen months of prior coverage under a group health or government insurance plan

- You are a resident of the state in which you are applying

- You are not eligible for coverage under a group health plan, Medicare, or Medicaid

- You have no break in health insurance coverage for sixty-three or more days from the termination of your previous insurance

Monthly costs of these plans can vary and they can have relatively expensive annual deductibles with high premium costs. Some plans are secondary to Medicare and have no deductible. For more information, contact your state's insurance commission.

Basic Health Insurance Plans

Basic health insurance plans are available in some states if you meet the criteria for low income. Premium costs are very moderate, but due to the recessionary economic conditions in many states the availability of these plans can be limited, or waiting lists can be exceptionally long.

What If You Run Out of Options?

In some instances, due to eligibility criteria, financial status, extended wait lists, and so on, you may run out of health insurance options. Having MS, it is critical that you maintain your medical care and medication. Outside of borrowing money from your friends and family to pay for your medical coverage (remember, you are a very worthwhile cause!), you may need to seek treatment at a city or county public health clinic. If you are a veteran, you may qualify for treatment at a Veterans Administration hospital if you meet various criteria.

Some of these clinical settings may be able to provide you with medication, but this is likely to be only on a short-term basis. It may be of greatest benefit for you to apply directly to the pharmaceutical maker of the medication recommended by your physician (see company contact information in table 1.1 in chapter 1.) Different pharmaceutical companies will have grant programs at varying times. Some university MS clinics will be evaluating different medications in clinical research programs. If you are enrolled in such a program and a medication is effective for you within this program, it's likely that the pharmaceutical company will maintain you on the medication regimen, at no additional cost if necessary. Contact the National Multiple Sclerosis Society (NMSS) or its local chapter for more ideas in this area. In terms of receiving adequate medical treatment, tenacity and creativity go a long way. Enlist your friends, spouses, and significant others in this effort.

Health Insurance Pros and Cons

If you find yourself in a health insurance coverage crisis, here is a worksheet to use while you consider and review the different avenues of health insurance coverage that may meet your needs.

Note: You are likely to be more successful in receiving Social Security support if you follow the
es outlined in chapter 11.

URING MEDICAID FOR LONG-TERM CARE:
OF AN INCOME CAP TRUST

re in need of long-term care, nursing home costs and other forms of long-term assisted living can
tely drain your available income and savings. However, if you engage a lawyer to establish an
cap trust and thus take control of any income or savings that you have in excess of the amount
uld require you to be cut off from Medicaid, you can then qualify for Medicaid. Your excess funds
held in the trust and can be used only for special needs, e.g., a motorized scooter, special trans-
ion costs, an enlarged computer screen, a voice-activated computer, a cell phone due to medical
ity, and so on. Your available income up to the amount of the Medicaid cutoff will be for a personal
allowance, a community spouse income allowance, and medical needs not covered by Medicaid in
ursing home. The state will pay the rest of the monies to the nursing facility.

Obviously, the purpose of the income cap trust is to change the manner in which Medicaid assesses
available income by eliminating from consideration the income that would render you ineligible for
icaid. If you are unable to pay for long-term care, this may be the best avenue for you to pursue.
e: It is important to understand, however, that after your death the state becomes entitled to the
eeds from the trust. You will not be able to leave monies to your spouse, significant other, or your
dren. If you feel mentally capable, you may be able to establish this trust for yourself and make
sions about it. In other cases, an attorney or conservator (spouse, significant other, or family friend)
nt be the best choice for the trustee. Regulations on these trusts vary by state and it can be helpful to
sult with an attorney familiar with state law. You should also contact your state Medicaid agency. (See
Resources section in the back for a Web address.)

If you have no assets (less than $2,000) and minimal income, you could be eligible for Medicaid for
g-term care support. When your need for physical care is less substantial and you do not require
enty-four-hour physical care, you can seek community home-care support through your state health
d human resources agency. Through this mechanism you can be supported in your home until twenty-
ur-hour residential care might be needed. This involves a state waiver to allow use of Medicaid funds for
-home care. Financial eligibility requirements, although similar to long-term care, will vary support
mewhat from state to state.

STRUCTURING YOUR PENSION AND RETIREMENT SAVINGS

ou may be in a position in which you have significant savings, an IRA/Keogh Plan, a pension payout, and
o forth—basically a significant amount of money that must be used wisely. You'll need to consider
tructuring how you'll use these funds based not only upon the amount of funds available, but also upon
your medical prognosis. If your physician's prognosis for your capacities over time is relatively "stable" and
you need to depend on a steady income stream, you might want to consider purchasing a lifetime annuity
guaranteeing a stable income.

WORKSHEET 18:   MAINTAINING MEDICAL CARE

1. Somehow maintain last employer's insurance

    Pro(s) _____

    Con(s) _____

2. Change job, use HIPAA to secure new insurance

    Pro(s) _____

    Con(s) _____

3. Use COBRA to extend benefits from last employer

    Pro(s) _____

    Con(s) _____

4. Apply for insurance from state insurance pool for high-risk individuals

    Pro(s) _____

    Con(s) _____

5. Apply for state basic health plan for low-income people

    Pro(s) _____

    Con(s) _____

6. Seek medical care through county/city health clinics or the Veterans Administration

    Pro(s) _____

    Con(s) _____

7. Seek available medication through pharmaceutical company grants/university research programs

    Pro(s) _____

    Con(s) _____

Evaluating Your Health Insurance Policy

As many readers already know, health insurance policies can vary widely in coverage and restrictions. Working with the following worksheet should help you understand some critical aspects of your health insurance:

WORKSHEET 19:   EVALUATING YOUR HEALTH CARE POLICY

What is the extent of the critical services that you need covered and how much is the deductible for each treatment or on an annual basis? _____

_____

What is your co-pay structure? _____

_____

What are the specifics of your pharmacy coverage? _____

_____

Are there financial limits on length of hospitalization, tests, number of physicians' visits, surgery, and other specialized services? _____

_____

Are certain medical interventions specifically excluded or simply not covered? _____

_____

What are your choices regarding the providers you can see? _____

_____

Long-Term Care

If you anticipate a need for long-term care, there is another type of policy that you should explore. That is, you should try to secure a policy with a fixed premium and an inflation rider that adjusts the benefit rate to the time of use. All levels of care should be covered in this policy and reimbursement should be provided for the actual cost of services versus a fixed sum. Look for policies with short waiting periods for coverage (100 days or less) and offering four or more years of nursing home coverage. For many of you with MS, long-term care coverage very obviously falls into the category of luxury. For others, however—those who are alone or don't wish to impose the burden of their care on their families, and can afford it—long-term care can be a very worthwhile option.

MAINTAINING YOUR INCOME STREAM

Aside from your health insurance coverage concerns, there are m... considerations that are important for you. These include how you handl... your short- and perhaps long-term disability income, the amount you... Social Security benefits, your pension structure, and the amount tha... Individual Retirement Account (IRA) or Keogh program.

If you are not working, your daily expenditures will decrease, but, o... salary. For most mid-career persons who leave work, their income strean... short/long-term disability, pension or IRA/Keogh, some savings, and, even... that may take some time to secure (see chapter 11 on the application p... strategies to employ when applying).

DEBT CONSOLIDATION/REDUCTION

If you have significant debt, your first step should be to reduce your high-i... credit card debts and personal loans. This would involve paying off as much... transferring to new credit cards at lower introductory rates, or negotiating *exte...* *increasing the interest.* You simply don't want to be in the position of paying the m... monthly payment amounts with no substantial payments to the balance of the... you have many debts, it might be wise for you to consult a credit counseling s... consolidate your debt into a payment to be distributed by them to your credit... such as chapter 7 liquidation bankruptcies or chapter 13 repayment plans, are a... or legal aid association, but most creditors will agree to a fixed nominal pa... significant losses if you choose the bankruptcy option. Under the Bush Admi... reform bill, S. 256, however, Chapter 7 "start fresh" bankruptcies will be... requirements and you will need a lawyer. Chapter 13 requires payment of some de... according to the debtor's resources. You will be required to see a credit counselor... prior to discharge of debt under either chapter. Of course, bankruptcy should be... because it will have a severe impact on your ability to secure credit or financing in th...

SOCIAL SECURITY PROGRAMS

If you have a substantive work background, Social Security Disability Income (SSDI) is... a monthly subsidy if you meet eligibility criteria. To obtain SSDI, your disability must... what is called "substantial gainful activity," meaning that you earn less than $830 per... month if you are blind). These amounts will be periodically adjusted upward. You... evaluated earnings by having an Impairment-Related Work Expenses (IWRE) plan.

Supplemental Security Income (SSI) is available for individuals who haven't work... required number of work credits. Your SSI payment is reduced dollar for dollar with any... (unless you can reduce income due to your work-related expenses on a Plan for Achievi... [PASS] plan). If you are eligible to receive SSI, you will immediately become eligibl...

---

benefits.
procedu...

SEC U...
USE...

If you...
compl...
incom...
that w...
will b...
porta...
neces...
needs...
the n...

your...
Med...
Not...
proc...
chil...
deci...
mig...
con...
the...

lor...
tw...
an...
fo...
in...
so...

If you have chronic progressive MS and you anticipate the need to seek nursing home care under Medicaid, you might be in a "spend down" mode in relation to your expenses. It's important to remember that if you meet the IRS code definition for disability under Section 72 (because you are unable to work due to a disability that would result in death, or of long and indefinite duration), the 10-percent penalty will be waived for prematurely taking funds out of your employer's retirement fund. This does not apply, however, to your personal IRA/Keogh plan. With your physician providing you with a medical prognosis, it can be very helpful to discuss options for optimal distribution or investment of your retirement savings with an accountant or certified financial planner (CFP). Ideally, you should consult with an independent CFP at an hourly rate.

INCOME TAX CONSIDERATIONS

If your MS is severe enough to meet the IRS definition of disability, you will be eligible for the Elderly and Permanently and Totally Disabled Tax Credit. If you are under sixty-five, you must have retired on disability leave for permanent or total disability before the end of the tax year in which you retired. This 15-percent credit (which lowers your actual tax bill by 15 percent) is applied after subtracting all nontaxable government benefits.

It is important that all medical expenses exceeding 7.5 percent of your adjusted gross income (AGI) are documented, because such expenses are tax deductible. This obviously relates to direct medical care and medication, but other disability-related costs must also be considered. That is, include attendant care/travel for medical care (check specific allowances here), home modifications, the need for extra living space for an attendant, or various kinds of assistive technology. That technology can involve a wide range of aids from enlarged computer screens to voice-activated software that can be directly linked to improving your functional capacity in your own home.

Social Security IRWE and PASS Plans

If you are on Social Security Disability Income (SSDI) and wish to work part-time, the cost of Impairment-Related Work Expenses (IRWEs) can be used as an offset to your income, e.g., the cost of a driver to get you, the worker, to your job or of an air-conditioned system that enables you to function in your office.

If the costs of these "assists" on a monthly basis reduce your salary to under $830 a month, you are not considered as being involved in substantial gainful activity (SGA). It should be noted that, when using your nine-month Trial Work Period (a time-limited period in which you can earn in excess of $830 a month to explore your work capacity), you are also not considered as being involved in SGA. If you are receiving Supplemental Security Income (SSI), a Plan for Achieving Self-Support (PASS) can be developed which similarly offsets income with the costs of the ancillary services and assistive technologies that enable you to work. You should consult a state vocational rehabilitation counselor or advocate from a local multiple sclerosis association who can help you develop these plans. Or you can hire a specialist who will do the same.

It is also of interest that certain subsidies received for being a volunteer, e.g., an Americorps (former Vista program) volunteer, are not considered taxable income. You may be able to secure an Americorps position, e.g., a literary counselor in a secondary school, and receive a subsidy of approximately $850 per month that will not be considered substantial gainful activity. Read Kurt's story below to see how this works.

Kurt's Story

Kurt is a fifty-two-year-old former loan officer who can no longer work full-time. He applied for and receives SSDI, but he is still able to work part-time doing loan processing.

Kurt's SSDI: $1,275 per month

Part-time earnings in mortgage processing: $1,400

Cost of driver/aide (Impairment-Related Work Expenses): $775 per month

Reduced Earnings = $775; Total: = $1900 monthly take-home

The cost of an aide who helps him get ready for work and drives him to a suburban bank is $775. This reduces his taxable earnings due to the IRWE as in the example. Kurt enjoys his work and, although the driver is expensive, he enjoys the flexible access to a ride to work and not having to deal with public transportation.

FINANCIAL PLANNING

Before you meet with your accountant or financial planner, it is critical to accurately and realistically assess your financial picture. It's sort of like putting all your cards on the table. You might use the same form as shown in worksheet 20 below or another, but you should do one for your current situation (especially if you're still working), one if you leave work, and another that would estimate your financial position five to ten years from today.

On worksheet 20, potential resources, such as your home equity, are listed at the end of the Assets section because these can be tapped for cash resources, if needed. As an example, in the case of a house in which you have significant equity, you might use a line of credit on your house or a reverse mortgage that can provide a monthly income stream from a bank. The bank will collect the loaned amount later at the time when your house is sold. In this manner, you may be enabled to stay in your house as long as possible.

When completing the worksheet, include your spouse's or significant other's income if that applies as an asset. The issue is how much money is available to you or how much could you "tap" on a *monthly* basis. Think outside the box; for example, could you rent out a room in your home? Would your income/available funds be so low that you might become be eligible for Section 8 housing or other low-cost housing? Are there certain staples that you can get every month from a local food bank? It's important to be candid with your financial planner during your discussion of your options.

WORKSHEET 20:   ASSESSING YOUR FINANCIAL STATUS

Current Monthly Assets

TAXABLE INCOME

Salary/Wages   _____

Dividends/Interest   _____

Other Taxable Income   _____

Alimony   _____

Business Earnings   _____

Property/Room Rental Income   _____

IRA/Keogh Payments   _____

Annuity/Pension Payments   _____

NONTAXABLE INCOME

Social Security (after potential   _____
application of IRWE/PASS Plan)

Disability Benefits   _____

Other Nontaxable Income   _____

Other Nontaxable Subsidy   _____

Total Monthly Available Income   _____

Assets That Could Be Used

Stocks   _____

Savings/CD   _____

Bonds   _____

Current Equity in Home/Reverse   _____

Mortgage Availability

Money Market   _____

Checking   _____

Life Insurance (Net Cash Value)   _____

Automobile (Net Value)   _____

Inheritance   _____

Other Net Assets   _____
(e.g., art, furniture, etc.)

Total Available Equity   _____

Monthly Expenditures

Mortgage/Rent   _____
(average, not covered)

Auto Payment   _____

Credit Card Payments

_____   _____

_____   _____

_____   _____

Home Insurance   _____

Medical Insurance   _____

Life Insurance   _____

Medical Expenditures   _____
(average, not covered)

Dental Expenses   _____
(average, not covered)

Eye Care Expenses   _____

Support of Children   _____

Tuition Costs   _____

Mandatory Expenses

  Food   _____

  Electricity   _____

  Phone(s)   _____

  Water/Sewer   _____

  Other   _____

Total Monthly Expenses   _____

In relation to the monthly expenses chart, it is important to assess whether any monthly expenses could be eliminated or drastically reduced by tapping home equity or other resources, specifically credit-card debt and interest payments. Based on your eligibility, could you also reduce your costs by obtaining food stamps or using a local food bank? Is your life insurance plan critical or would a different form of coverage, such as term insurance, be less costly? Would a different car be more economical? Again, be creative. As one of our clients noted, "I am doing well financially because I am honest with myself and budget!" He has secured SSDI, pays only $200 a month for a big, pleasant apartment on Section 8 housing, and does some part-time bookkeeping at home earning several hundred dollars a month. He plans, works, and lives within his means.

Conclusion

We hope that this chapter encourages you to tackle some of your tough financial issues if you haven't already done so. Seek help from financial planners, or reputable credit assistance agencies, local multiple sclerosis associations, and other helping professionals whenever possible. It's important to try to secure as much control over your finances as you can. It's important because difficulties or actual chaos in this area can be a significant stressor or emotional drain, not only on yourself, but on your significant others, as well. We send our very best to you as you successfully take control of your life in this important area of your finances.

CHAPTER 10

Help with Cognitive Problems: Using Neuropsychological Information Effectively

David C. Clemmons, Ph.D., C.R.C.

COGNITIVE PROBLEMS PEOPLE WITH MS OFTEN HAVE

According to research in this area, it seems that a substantial proportion of those with multiple sclerosis (MS) will have at least some significant cognitive difficulties within a range of 45 to 65 percent (Rao 1995). There appears to be a pattern to these difficulties. Some areas of ability remain relatively strong, while others may get weaker. For instance, although you may do well on standard intelligence tests (IQ tests), you may have other cognitive problems. You may also continue to have very good language skills, especially if you've had college education or professional or technical kinds of jobs. Because of this ability, it can sometimes be difficult for you to recognize that you are having cognitive difficulties, or how important they are. If you have some "unclear" cognitive concerns, this can be confusing not only to you, but to those with whom you interact.

Note that some people with MS have few or no cognitive problems. For example, if most of your multiple sclerosis lesions are located in your spinal cord, you might have difficulty with muscle control, but you might not have any problems at all with your cognitive abilities. A full neuropsychological assessment should be performed.

Worksheet 21 presents an overview of the areas that may be affected. I've put asterisks (*) next to the four areas that can be especially vulnerable if you have MS. Checklist 11 explains these four areas in greater detail.

WORKSHEET 21:   SEVEN AREAS COMMONLY ASSESSED IN NEUROPSYCHOLOGICAL TEST BATTERIES

Sensorimotor Ability. Do the areas of the brain responsible for controlling the body's muscles function efficiently? Does the brain efficiently process input from the sensory organs? (This is technically not a cognitive function but it's important to measure sensorimotor function to make sure that the brain is getting good information from the outside world.)

Attention and Concentration. *Attention* is the ability to focus on individual stimuli. *Concentration* is the ability to maintain that focus in the presence of distractions for an extended period of time.

Memory.* Visual-spatial memory; verbal memory; long- and short-term memory; incidental memory versus memory for rehearsed or practiced items. *Short-term memory* is important for learning new material and efficient functioning. *Incidental memory,* which is memory for things (e.g., in the environment) that did not seem important at the time, is also important for efficient functioning. *Verbal memory* is memory for material that is heard. *Visual-spatial memory* helps in remembering locations and in some types of learning.

Language Ability. The ability to understand language and to use it to express ideas.

Spatial Ability.* The ability to deal with two- and three-dimensional formats, perceive whole/part relationships, and perceive field-background relationships.

Cognitive Efficiency.* The ability to perform simultaneous tasks efficiently, or to perform tasks in the presence of competing stimuli. The ability to screen out extraneous stimuli.

Executive Function.* This refers to the ability to deal with abstractions, and to do problem solving, self-regulation, and initiate plans.

The areas most frequently compromised may be evident in the different types of memory, but very much less so in the case of the other functions. When you review the short list of cognitive concerns in checklist 11, below, it can be helpful to check in with your family and friends to get their opinions.

---

* These functions are frequently compromised if you have MS (Clemmons et al. 2004).

Checklist 11: The Short List of Cognitive Concerns

1. Since you've had MS, have you noticed increased problems with short-term memory? _____

2. Is it more difficult for you now to do several things at once and to process them quickly? _____

3. Are you having difficulty in problem solving, planning, initiating, and evaluating your activities? Is it difficult to think through your problems? _____

Again, you might want to review these questions with a family member or friend to get their perspective!

Difficulties with Memory

People with MS frequently say things about their memory like the following two statements:

In school, I always used to be able to learn things quickly. Now it seems like I can't remember anything.

I can't make up my mind whether my spouse just doesn't listen carefully, or whether he really has some kind of memory problem.

Memory is a very important ability. If you have difficulty in this area, you're likely to have difficulty with social interactions, job performance, and even the basic activities of daily living. People with MS frequently have difficulty with memory. Even when testing demonstrates that someone's memory appears to be within the average range, a very common complaint is that the person's memory doesn't seem to be as efficient as it once was.

It's very unusual for problems with memory to involve things learned long ago. Memory for skills well-learned, events in personal history, and knowledge developed in the past is often relatively stable. What seems to be affected most is memory for very recent events. If you have MS, often the many new experiences and interactions we all have every day become harder to remember. This, of course, can interfere with learning new tasks or following through with plans or commitments. Memory function can be especially affected if new learning situations involve information that changes frequently. Busy or noisy learning situations can also interfere with your ability to retain new memories.

The busy parent. Consider a busy parent, one who works half- or full-time, drives the kids to soccer practice, shops, prepares meals, breaks up children's arguments, and so on during the course of a busy day. Because this person is operating in an environment that constantly changes, her short-term memory abilities are very important. Missing a business report deadline or forgetting an important soccer match causes problems for everyone involved. Not remembering a spouse's business dinner or a slumber party for the kids' friends can create friction in the household and embarrassment or self-esteem problems for the parent.

However, there is some good news about these memory concerns. Some research suggests that the problem is not so much with the actual learning part of making a memory, but with retrieving memories that have already been stored (Rao et al. 1984). For example, you may do better on memory tests when you have memory cues, or where you have some structure that helps you to remember. This suggests that your memory problems may be problems of retrieving memories.

This is better news than it would be if the memories had not been formed, and stored, in the first place. It also suggests that structuring situations and providing memory cues can make your memory function more efficiently, and that memory practice and overlearning information may be a useful strategy. For instance, suppose you want to remember a work task such as the steps involved in bringing up a certain computer program. It can be useful to repetitively bring up the program, close it down, bring it up again, and so on, until you can do it automatically.

Difficulties with Multitasking/Processing Information

"Nowadays, I just get swamped by the multiple tasks I have to do that I used to field so easily at my job." This is a very common report from people with MS who have cognitive problems. It is an example of multitasking challenges. Because multitasking involves processing many tasks efficiently, this ability is also referred to as *cognitive efficiency*. Complaints of falling behind, having difficulty keeping up with the flow, or becoming easily distracted may become predictable for you if you are having difficulty with cognitive efficiency or multitasking. You may find yourself processing information much more slowly than you used to, before you had MS. You may no longer enjoy the busy or even hectic pace of your job.

As stated in the discussion about memory above, you can be operating less efficiently than before. This can be a very distressing situation. You may be feeling overwhelmed by all the details of daily life, but still fondly remember having efficiently organized your family's affairs while holding down a busy job. Understandably, you may feel a sense of loss and frustration. Equally distressing may be the feeling that you "should" be keeping up and that your difficulties suggest you are lazy or disinterested.

You might want to reread the example of a busy parent's day a few paragraphs above. If you do read it again, you will see that this, too, could be cited as an example of someone having difficulty with multitasking abilities. Stop and think about this for a minute because this is an important point. Often, people don't have problems in just one area of cognitive functioning. The problems are likely to be interactive: that is, problems with multitasking cause difficulties with remembering things, and problems remembering things cause less efficiency with multitasking.

You can see how confusing this might become, unless there is a way to identify and measure one's cognitive abilities. The interactive nature of many cognitive problems, that is, how they affect each other, is even more important in the next area to be discussed: executive functioning.

Difficulty with Executive Functioning

Difficulties with executive functioning often give rise to comments like these:

John used to be such a go-getter. Now he hardly ever initiates anything. He makes plans, but he never acts on them, and he seems stuck.

I don't think Sally means to be impolite, but sometimes she doesn't make good social decisions. She says she is just trying to be friendly, but sometimes people feel her behavior is inappropriate or that she can't figure out social situations.

Much research and experience suggests that "executive functioning" is an area in which many people with MS experience at least some difficulties. There are many aspects to executive functioning. *Executive abilities* is the name given to the abilities we use to run our lives effectively, to make good decisions, and to organize our lives. Like a good executive, these abilities help us to manage our affairs and to stay organized. Executive abilities are also important to social problem solving and maintaining socially appropriate behavior. Abstraction, the ability to receive input from the environment and come to general conclusions, is an important executive function. Difficulties with abstraction lead to poor problem solving and poor decision making. Also, weaknesses in this area may make it challenging to appreciate another's point of view.

As the term "executive" suggests, these are also the abilities that are important to initiating and regulating behaviors. Problems in this area may lead to problems with impulsive behavior or to difficulty in following through with commitments and responsibilities. Previously energetic and dynamic persons may become less organized and self-directed. These changes may be misunderstood by family members and friends. They can be wrongly interpreted as laziness or carelessness.

In addition, when you are having problems with executive functioning, if you find yourself on a wrong course, it can be very difficult to correct and redirect the direction in which you are headed. Unfortunately, as problems with executive functioning increase, it is not uncommon to have greater difficulty understanding the nature of a problem. You may not even realize that there is a serious problem. Because of this cognitive deficit, it may also become more difficult to understand difficulties with spouses, or significant others and associates. This, in turn, is likely to increase the misunderstanding and difficulty with communication.

Again, as discussed above, cognitive abilities are often interactive. If your other abilities, such as multitasking and memory are less efficient, your executive function will suffer, too. Thus, executive functioning may get worse if you have to retrieve information quickly or you must process large amounts of complex information. Success at tasks like operating a complicated computer program or keeping up with the changing needs and moods of children depends on an efficient memory, the ability to multitask, and efficient executive functioning.

IDENTIFY YOUR COGNITIVE PROBLEMS WITH NEUROPSYCHOLOGICAL TESTING

When cognitive abilities are being discussed, you might think of IQ tests or intelligence tests. IQ tests can be useful to you in terms of understanding some of your strengths and weaknesses, but they have many limitations. Unfortunately, they don't measure many of the areas of cognitive ability that are important in everyday life. Also, they were not designed to measure the kinds of problems you may experience with MS. With MS, you can have cognitive difficulties and may still score reasonably well on IQ tests because of old verbal learning, such as vocabulary. Consequently, tests that are more sensitive to specific cognitive problems (i.e., memory) and *new learning capacities* are a better choice than IQ tests or other standard tests used to measure intelligence. These are called neuropsychological tests.

Neuropsychological tests are designed to measure many different kinds of brain abilities. Because we use our brains in order to adapt to our living environment, these abilities are often called *adaptive abilities*. Many different adaptive abilities can be measured by neuropsychological testing. These include such diverse abilities as attention and concentration, different types of memory function, multitasking, problem solving, and several other important abilities.

Look for Your Areas of Strength

It's important to know that although neuropsychological tests are usually given only when people suspect a problem, these tests can be very useful for identifying areas of strength, as well as areas in which there may be deficits. Because of this, they're quite useful in planning. Here are some ways in which neuropsychological testing can provide you with useful information or a basis for making plans. They can help you to:

1. Identify your cognitive strengths and weaknesses.

2. Make better educational and vocational choices.

3. Choose an appropriate type of counseling or psychotherapy.

4. Identify environments and interventions that will accommodate your limitations successfully.

5. Make decisions about your ability to successfully perform activities like financial management, driving, or independent living.

6. Solve your specific concerns regarding "reasonable accommodations," diminished work performance, forgetting, difficulties with problem solving, and improving your communication skills.

7. Establish information about your level of capacity for Social Security or disability pension considerations.

These are just a few of the possible uses of neuropsychological data. Additionally, information from a neuropsychological test battery sometimes provides you with important positive feedback. You may experience a sense of satisfaction when neuropsychological testing points out your areas of relative strength and ability. Even if you are aware that you are having some type of cognitive difficulties, these concerns may be vague and poorly defined. You may feel a sense of relief and validation once your cognitive problems are more accurately defined in measurable terms. Some of your problems that you suspect are cognitive in their origin may, in fact, be more related to physical fatigue or depression. Neuropsychological test results can often put some of your concerns to rest.

The Limitations of Neuropsychological Testing

It's also important to understand that neuropsychological tests do not always provide an accurate picture of a person's functioning. From a statistical standpoint they are very accurate instruments. For instance, if the researcher administers the neuropsychological test battery to one hundred people, there is a strong likelihood that the battery will be able to identify which of these people have difficulty with cognitive functioning and which do not. When a neuropsychologist administers the same battery to a single person, however, many other factors, such as fatigue, motivation, pain, stress, and depression, can affect that person's performance. Cultural differences and many other factors also can affect scores.

Another problem that can occur is sometimes the neuropsychologist doesn't have a good medical or psychosocial history for the person being tested. When that happens, the neuropsychologist may not make an accurate analysis of the meaning of the test results because of the missing information. Finally, sometimes someone might do poorly on the tests, but still perform life activities well due to years of practice.

All of this is just another way to say that you have to be careful about believing that test results always measure your actual capacities accurately. For this reason, it is best to use the results of a neuro-psychological evaluation to form a "best guess," or an hypothesis about someone's cognitive functioning. Then, we try to see whether the "best guess" is useful in explaining problems you may be experiencing in your daily activities and in dealing with your environment.

In vocational programs, for example, it is quite common to use the neuropsychological evaluation to make a best guess about which types of jobs are most likely to accommodate specific difficulties. Then, a two- to three-month internship or unpaid work experience can be developed with a local company to make sure that the best guess from the evaluation really does match the person's work capacities. We call this experience "community-based" because it is done in a real-life situation, instead of a counseling office or within an institution. This community-based assessment is often supported by state rehabilitation agencies as discussed in chapter 7. (See also appendix C.)

CHOOSING AND WORKING WITH A NEUROPSYCHOLOGIST

If you decide to get neuropsychological testing, this section will help you to choose the right person. It helps to be a good consumer in order to ensure that you are tested by someone who can use and interpret the tests correctly. A *neuropsychologist* is a licensed psychologist with specific training in giving and interpreting neuropsychological tests. Many other psychologists use neuropsychological tests occasionally, but they don't have the comprehensive training that a neuropsychologist has received. Also, neuropsycho-logical tests are not controlled by neuropsychologists. Any psychologist who wants to buy and use them can do so. Because of this, you will need a plan for choosing the right professional.

Here are some tips that will be useful for choosing and for working with a neuropsychologist.

You have a right to request a résumé from any neuropsychologist with whom you are considering working. This résumé should list the psychologist's education as well as other kinds of training. A person who is practicing as a neuropsychologist should have a degree in psychology. Specific training in using neuropsychological tests is also a must. There should also be supervised training after the person receives a Ph.D. This is often called an "internship." Many neuropsychologists also have an advanced certification that is called a "diplomate certification." This certification, as issued by the American Board of Professional Psychology, is also referred to as an "ABPP certification." Neuropsychologists who have ABPP certification are likely to have a very solid preparation to practice as neuropsychologists, although some very good ones have not yet taken this examination.

Word-of-mouth. This can be a very effective way to determine if a neuropsychologist has provided services that have proved useful to other people. It would be helpful if you could find individuals who could give you references for neuropsychologists with whom they have worked, e.g., through support groups. Agencies such as local multiple sclerosis associations may be useful places to get this kind of information or to meet people who have had satisfying experiences with neuropsychologists.

Many state, county, or city mental health organizations have listings of neuropsychologists. You can look for these lists through psychological or neuropsychological associations, medical school departments of rehabilitation medicine or neurology, and university psychology departments. Other local neuro-psychologists may have all their pertinent information available for viewing on their Web sites.

State rehabilitation agencies may provide neuropsychological testing for people who qualify for services. Although state agency personnel may be in the habit of referring to specific practitioners for getting neuropsychological testing, it is still important to be a good consumer. Recent legislation and policy trends emphasize "client choice" policies.

Make Sure You Get a Personalized Report

Finding the neuropsychologist with whom you want to work is only half of the job. There are two more tasks you need to do:

1. First, it's important to make sure that the neuropsychologist has enough medical vocational/educational (transcripts), and social information from your account of your history to make accurate judgments about what your test scores mean. As mentioned above, just having the test scores is not always useful. They mean a lot more when they are used with an understanding of the person's medical and social history. For instance, if you were raised in another country, or you have hand tremors, you may score differently than other people. It's important to make sure the neuropsychologist gets this kind of information so that the report can be as accurate as possible.

    It is also important to try to remember whether you've had psychological or educational evaluations in the past. If this was the case, try to make sure that the neuropsychologist gets copies. Usually, it's more useful for the neuropsychologist to be able to read this kind of information in its original form. Also, a review of any nationally standardized educational test scores from your high school and/or college transcript can be very helpful.

2. Second, it's important to provide the neuropsychologist with a letter that has specific questions to be answered. This is also a way to make sure that your report is a personalized report. Imagine for a minute that you are a neuropsychologist writing a report. If the person whom you tested had not given you some specific questions to answer, you may have to guess at which recommendations would be most helpful. Remember the old saying from the early computer programmers: "Garbage in, garbage out"? The higher the quality of your background information and your questions, the more useful the neuropsychologist's report will be. You can use worksheet 22, below, to prepare the questions to include in your letter.

WORKSHEET 22:   QUESTIONS FOR YOUR NEUROPSYCHOLOGIST

Examples:

1. In a summary, can you tell me what are my specific cognitive assets and what are my specific deficits?

2. Can you help me figure out a way of talking about my disability-related concerns with others?

3. Do I have the ability to do well in a technical graduate degree/program? Is further academic training in my best interest? Would I do better in on-the-job training?

4. My performance at work has gone down steadily for the past four months. Can you suggest some procedures or equipment that might help me to improve my job performance?

Your Questions for the Neuropsychologist

Of course, the questions above are just examples. But after reading them, you should have some idea of the kinds of questions you want to ask the neuropsychologist. Also, be sure to get some input from your family and friends. They may come up with some important questions to ask that you might overlook.

1. _____

2. _____

3. _____

You can probably think of other questions to ask because the suggestions above are just generalized examples that different people might use. It's more likely that you will receive a more personalized report from the neuropsychologist if you generate your own questions.

If you have difficulty coming up with questions, think about your life since the onset of MS. Reviewing a typical day (or week) in your life since you began living with MS, and thinking about the difficulties you've been dealing with will probably help you generate specific questions to ask the neuropsychologist.

If you're living with a spouse or significant other, it would be a good idea to make sure that his or her point of view is also given to the neuropsychologist. Sometimes, people we know and care for have very different ideas about the nature of our relationship with them and about what kinds of interpersonal problems exist. For example, a spouse may have questions about how MS affects the couple relationship or he or she may disagree with you about how to best help you.

If you must live with and get along with a life partner, it is a good idea to make sure that your partner has a chance to ask questions too. Sometimes, it's a good idea for each person involved in a relationship to write separate referral letters to the neuropsychologist to ensure that each has the privacy needed to feel safe about honestly saying what they think about the situation. If you live with a life partner, it would be an excellent idea to discuss this suggestion with that person.

In reading the paragraph above, you may have seen a possible problem arising if more than one person becomes involved in writing a referral letter. Usually, the more information a psychologist gets, the better the report will be. When more than one person is involved, however, it's also very important to make sure the person being tested is not made to feel uncomfortable.

If you are the person to receive the testing, you probably understand that the report will be more useful if your life partner also contributes to the questions to be asked. Even so, it would be entirely natural if you were uncomfortable about this. Before you invite other people to include their questions in a letter, you should talk to them about your possible concerns. There may be times when it is not a good idea for anyone but the person being tested to ask the referral questions. Because people are so different, the question of whether other people should be involved in asking questions of the neuropsychologist has to be decided on an individual basis. Except in unusual situations, the person being tested should have the right to make this decision. If there is a conflict, talk to your physician, social worker, counselor, or an advocate from a local MS association.

Some Examples and Hints on Writing Referral Letters

You probably don't write referral letters every day, so we are providing some examples of shared information about some of the questions to ask. First, here is how part of a letter from a worker with memory and multitasking problems might look:

I seem to have more and more difficulty learning new procedures and keeping up with the rest of the staff at work. Sometimes I'm exhausted by the end of the day. My memory seems to be a big part of the problem. I think that I can manage if I can take some of the work home, but I need to learn some ways to become more efficient at work. I also need some ways to help my husband understand that I can handle this on my own.

This person's spouse might also write a referral letter, which might include the following concerns:

I am worried because my wife is working harder at her job, but seems to be overwhelmed with it. She often brings work home overnight. She's worried that if she asks for an accommodation at her job that she will hurt her chances for a promotion. She has always been very independent. I'm worried that she thinks that she must be a high achiever for our family to love her. She can help others, but she has a hard time accepting help for herself.

As you can see, both of these people see the problem more or less in the same way, but with some different viewpoints. Can you spot an important counseling issue? The wife is concerned with demonstrating that she is still able to function independently, while her spouse is worried that she is cutting herself off from family support. This type of information can be quite useful to the neuropsychologist for suggesting possible counseling issues and strategies.

Generally, because neuropsychological testing is usually sought when specific problems are suspected, there may be a tendency to focus on problems rather than strengths. A good evaluation should point out areas of relative strength, and then suggest how these can be used in accommodation or communication strategies. It may be helpful to ask specifically for a discussion of your relative areas of strength and how these may be used to maximize your functioning in all of your life's tasks.

Operational Questions

Here's another important thing to think about. You can't expect the neuropsychologist to be an expert in every field. For this reason, it is usually more helpful to ask operational questions rather than general questions. In an *operational question,* you explain or define the object of your question. This makes the question more specific (and helpful).

If you are writing a letter to a neuropsychologist, and you want to know if a person will be able to cook meals, you might be tempted to ask the question this way: "Will James be able to cook meals independently?" This question seems simple enough, but other questions can arise from that seemingly simple question.

A more helpful way to phrase the question about cooking would go like this:

Do you think James will be able to follow a five- or six-step recipe by reading it from a cookbook? Will he have trouble if he has to cook more than one item at a time? Will he be able to cook efficiently if our two children are "helping" him? Should we be worried about safety issues, like his forgetting to turn off a burner?

Here's another example, this time about a job situation. Suppose you are helping your friend Sally write a question about how well she might do in retail sales. As above, you can just ask the question "How well do you think Sally will do in retail sales?" However, like the example about cooking, it would be more helpful to ask the question by telling the neuropsychologist exactly what your concerns are.

That is, it would be helpful for the neuropsychologist to know how many different essential tasks are required to do the job and how much time is spent on each task over the day. You could copy the job description developed by the company and send that. But even sending a job description developed by the company may be insufficient if the *essential functions* of the job are not clear and outlined as to the effort and the time frames involved. Some job descriptions are very generalized and don't really describe how the job is done. For job-related evaluations, the neuropsychologist should know the truly "critical" job tasks and the approximate number of hours involved in each. A work supervisor might be the best resource. Here are the key concerns that must be addressed in the referral letter to the neuropsychologist:

Elements for Referral Letter for Neuropsychological Testing

- Describe problems to be addressed. Be as specific as possible.

- Frame your questions operationally. (See Operational Questions above.)

- Include important medical and social history.

- Request a discussion of strengths as well as weaknesses.

- Request a discussion of accommodation strategies (e.g., procedural or assistive equipment).

- Request a discussion of specific counseling strategies, if appropriate.

- For job functioning concerns, have an accurate description of the job's key tasks and input from a supervisor or from the person being tested about which tasks are the most challenging.

- If possible, try to have input or separate letters from friends and significant others.

COSTS AND FUNDING SOURCES FOR NEUROPSYCHOLOGICAL ASSESSMENT

Neuropsychological testing can be expensive. A full neuropsychological evaluation can take most of a day, and, typically, involves the administration of both a neuropsychological test battery and a measure of intellectual functioning such as the Wechsler Adult Intelligence Scale-III (WAIS-III). It is also standard practice to administer some index of emotional functioning, such as the Minnesota Multiphasic Personality Inventory-2 (MMPI-2). A full neuropsychological evaluation can take an entire day of a psychologist's time or that of a psychometrist, who is an individual trained to administer, but not to interpret, neuropsychological tests. Review of background information, interview time, and report writing take additional time. Depending upon the circumstances and the geographic location, the cost of a comprehensive neuropsychological evaluation can range from $1,000 to $3,000 or even more.

If you want to obtain a neuropsychological evaluation, there are a number of options to consider before paying for it from your own pocket. Many medical plans will pay for a neuropsychological evaluation if it is requested by your physician. If this option is available, it would be desirable to involve the referring physician in generating the questions for the referral letter as discussed above.

Alternately, in a job situation, you may be able to request that your employer pay for a neuropsychological evaluation as part of a larger accommodation package in seeking technical assistance. The Americans with Disabilities Act (ADA) stipulates that many employers are responsible for seeking technical assistance in order to help individuals with medical conditions. Although it may feel threatening to disclose your medical condition, our experience suggests that often the energy involved in trying to mask problems with work performance, e.g., working longer hours, can be personally draining. Current rehabilitation legislation also makes it likelier that employers will try to provide you with reasonable accommodation if you request it.

If you are not working or if you are having difficulty maintaining your employment, the state rehabilitation agency is an option for providing neuropsychological evaluations, as well as access to assistive technology and other services. Individual counselors within the state rehabilitation system may or may not have specific training with respect to MS-related issues. For this reason, it may be desirable to provide a state vocational rehabilitation counselor with specific MS-related information, including information about the importance of obtaining a neuropsychological evaluation (see Clemmons et al. 2004 in the References section). In some cases, rather than waiting in a state of limbo, you may simply want to "bite the bullet" and pay for the evaluation yourself.

How Much Testing Do You Need? Are There Ways to Cut Costs?

The advantage of a full neuropsychological battery of tests is that it provides a comprehensive screening. Nevertheless, as suggested above, there appear to be some patterns seen in MS-related cognitive concerns. Because of this, much interest has been shown recently in developing brief neuropsychological screening batteries for MS that focus on these areas (Basso et al. 1996; Beatty et al. 1995; Rao, Leo, Bernardin, et al. 1991; Rao, Leo, Ellington, et al. 1991). Rao, especially, has studied a number of very brief screening batteries for use with people who have multiple sclerosis. As discussed above, these usually involve general areas such as short-term memory, multitasking ability and speed of information processing, and problem solving or executive functioning.

Building on the work of previous authors, Clemmons and colleagues (2004) developed an abbreviated neuropsychological screening battery for people with MS. This can be administered in approximately three hours and provides an estimate of intellectual functioning, as well as good coverage of the areas discussed above in addition to the functions of language, attention, and visual-spatial processing. We've used this battery to provide vocational and other types of counseling for people with MS seen in our vocational program. The battery is useful because it addresses the concerns of mid-career, semi-skilled and skilled professionals who seem to make up the bulk of the MS population.

It should be noted that brief test batteries may sacrifice the desirability of a broader evaluation of neuropsychological abilities to the advantage of saving money or time, while still being helpful. Someone with MS may have difficulties outside the three main areas first discussed. Nevertheless, there are times when it may be expedient to consider the use of a brief or abbreviated neuropsychological battery of tests due to the presenting clinical or time/cost considerations. This would be one of the issues you will want to discuss with the neuropsychologist with whom you are considering working.

The following is a short case history which can show you how all of this works together.

Case History: A Consultation with Nora

Nora, who has a master's degree in nursing, is a supervisor at an infirmary in a state penal institution. She was recently diagnosed with MS and is emotionally stressed. Nora and her husband had discussed not revealing her medical condition to the institution's administrative staff because she values her well-paid position. She is, however, experiencing memory problems and has received two write-ups by the institution's administrator for failing to attend a court hearing and for not scheduling the transfer of an inmate to the infirmary.

Nora knows she is having difficulties remembering nurses' absence requests and other administrative details and she is becoming less and less efficient. A job analysis indicates that her scheduling of nursing staff is a critical function and takes up almost half her work week. Another supervisor is encouraging her to seek disability consultation. With all the stress she is experiencing, Nora is becoming increasingly anxious and irritable at home, as well.

- Would you disclose to the administrator?

- Would you seek assistance, and how?

- How would you pay for the evaluation?

Outcome. After discussing all the issues with her husband, Nora talked to her supervisor about her need for accommodation and she scheduled a consultation with the state's disability services unit. This unit, with Nora's permission, sought assistance for assessment and accommodation recommendations from the neuropsychological and vocational rehabilitation unit within the neurology department of a local university. Nora's specific problems, as tested, were:

1. Some problems with her short-term verbal memory, and

2. Slow speed of information processing.

This meant that she was:

1. Having trouble remembering small but important daily facts, and

2. Her memory became even more inefficient when the work pace speeded up and became more hectic (which it often did).

The consultation team, with input from the Internet through West Virginia University's Job Accommodation Network (JAN), recommended a nurse-scheduling software package that reduced her scheduling demands from four hours a day to twenty-five minutes daily. With this extra time and with the aid of a personal digital assistant (PDA), she was able to keep quite organized and to maintain her job proficiency.

Previously, she had been trying to maintain the daily scheduling with a large wall chart and a pack of "yellow stickies." This consultation was kept as a confidential matter with disability services and the software costs were easily absorbed by the institution as part of regular office expenses. The institution's administrator was very enthusiastic about the improvement in Nora's functioning.

Although Nora and her husband did not write a referral letter about what they thought her problems were, the neuropsychologist was someone with a great deal of experience in this type of situation. In addition to the vocational rehabilitation recommendation about the software package to help Nora at her job, the neuropsychologist's report offered suggestions about how to manage the stress that she was experiencing and the growing friction at home. Due to a reduction in her workplace difficulties and the specific recommendations on how to deal with MS as a couple or a team, within a short time, Nora and her husband were happy to report they were experiencing much less stress in their relationship.

One of the reasons that Nora's case has a positive ending was that she was able to reach out for help relatively early. Counselors who provide social and vocational rehabilitation services for people with MS know that frequently it is difficult for people with MS to seek outside help. Sometimes, it can be uncomfortable to admit that a problem has grown large enough that you need to seek outside help, but many MS-related problems eventually do require specialized assistance. The good news is that this generally takes some of the burden off you, as an individual, and can provide new strategies for helping you to maximize your strengths and manage your limitations more effectively.

Conclusion

This chapter has reviewed some areas of neuropsychological ability that are important to life functioning, and it has offered you suggestions about finding and screening a qualified neuropsychologist. Neuropsychological testing can be seen either as targeting deficits or as defining the problems to be solved. For anyone who is worried about the possibility of losing some cognitive abilities, the tests can be perceived as threatening. For this reason, the emphasis in this chapter has been that this testing can be very helpful for identifying relative areas of strength. By identifying these areas of cognitive strength, the person who is having difficulties with vocational, social, or other areas of life functioning can begin to develop strategies for adaptation and accommodation. For the person with MS and that person's significant others or employers, early intervention can eliminate quite a lot of frustration and distress.

For those of you with MS, we hope that this discussion will encourage you to explore neuropsychological testing, if you think it might be helpful. For those of you who are significant others, this chapter has suggested ways for you to support and assist your loved one in finding appropriate testing and making the best use of it.

CHAPTER 11

Social Security Disability Insurance and Supplemental Security Income: How to Jump Through Hoops Without Stumbling

Peter H. D. McKee, J.D. and Alan Wittenburg, MSW

APPLYING FOR SOCIAL SECURITY?

For some of you, there may come a time when you conclude, often reluctantly, that you should apply for the disability benefits that are available from the Social Security Administration (SSA). Your decision to apply or not, and the impacts of your decision, can have long-range effects, both positive and negative. Legal, social, medical, vocational, financial, and emotional considerations must all be weighed when deciding whether to apply for Social Security disability benefits.

It might seem to you that applying for these benefits requires conquering seemingly insurmountable barriers of bureaucracy, delay, medical, and legal processing. However, with some knowledge of how the system works, and a strong sense of determination, along with the help of your friends, relatives, doctors, and other healthcare providers, this is an effort worth pursuing. What follows is intended to give you some starting tools to help you pursue your claim more effectively. Because this topic is vast, this chapter can provide only brief summaries of some of the important issues to consider when you apply for Social Security disability benefits. More information can be obtained from the resources listed below.

A Short List of Resources: Social Security Disability Claims

Social Security's own web site. See the Resources section in the back of the book. The link will connect you with an enormous collection of information about the rules, regulations, and other matters related to claims for both disability and retirement benefits.

The National Organization of Social Security Claimants' Representatives (NOSSCR). This nation-wide organization of lawyers and other advocates representing claimants with disability for Social Security benefits is a valuable resource. Many experienced lawyers handling these cases are members, and NOSSCR has a nationwide referral program to help you connect with an experienced practitioner. See the Resources section in the back of the book for contact information. You can contact NOSSCR at 560 Sylvan Avenue, Englewood Cliffs, NJ 06432, 800-431-2804, email NOSSCR@worldnet.att.net.

Be aware, however, that merely applying for disability benefits with the Social Security Administration, or simply carrying the diagnosis of multiple sclerosis, does *not* entitle you to an automatic grant of these benefits. These must be understood as merely the starting points in the undertaking of proving your eligibility for the available benefits. It is only with knowledge of the system and proof of the severity of your MS that you will have the best chance of winning your claim.

Note: *In the fall of 2003, the Commissioner of the Social Security Administration announced a comprehensive plan for major revisions of the way Social Security processes disability claims. These plans intend to alter many aspects of the applications and appeals process at all levels. The specific details of these plans, and when and how they will be implemented, are still being developed. Thus, some of what is described in the following materials may have changed to some degree in the past several years.*

BASIC FACTS YOU MUST KNOW ABOUT THE SOCIAL SECURITY DISABILITY SYSTEM

The Social Security Administration is a federal agency under the umbrella of the Department of Health and Human Services. This department administers two disability programs: Social Security Disability Income benefits (SSDI or Title II) and Supplemental Security Income (SSI or Title XVI).

Social Security Disability Insurance (SSDI) Benefits

Social Security's disability insurance program requires you to show that you are (1) *disabled* (as defined by Social Security) and (2) that you have worked and paid into the Social Security system by paying your insurance premiums. The way you paid your premiums was by having a work history and having paid your FICA taxes in the past. If you have never worked or paid FICA, you will not be eligible for these benefits, as you have not paid your insurance premiums.

Adult workers who seek SSDI must show that, from the date they first became disabled, they had paid into the Social Security system by working and paying FICA premiums on adequate earnings in five out of the last ten years (or twenty out of the last forty work quarters). Special rules apply to workers younger than thirty-one as to how many quarters of work they must have had to become eligible for coverage. Thus a claimant under age thirty-one must show that he or she worked and paid into the system for one-half of the quarters between the time the worker reached age twenty-one and the time the worker became disabled. For these reasons, *the date that you claim you became disabled can be critical in determining whether or not you have had sufficient earnings to be eligible for the insurance coverage.*

Supplemental Security Income (SSI)

Social Security also administers a second disability program called Supplemental Security Income (SSI) benefits. This program is similar to a public assistance disability program, in that you must show that you are disabled and that you have very little income and resources. To meet the financial eligibility requirements, you must show that you have no more than $2,000 in "non-exempt resources" as an individual, and that you have a very low income. The regulations regarding what resources are exempt are quite complex. As an example, such items as the house you live in and one car that you drive will not count toward the maximum resources you are allowed to have and still be eligible for SSI.

It is possible for you to receive both SSDI and SSI, depending on your benefit level when you are on Social Security. How much you will get per month if found eligible for Social Security Disability Income depends on your past work history. At the present time (2005), the maximum Social Security disability benefit payable to a single individual is approximately $1,825 per month. The maximum SSI benefit for an individual with no other income is approximately $579 per month. Annual cost-of-living raises are applied to these maximum amounts.

With both the SSDI and SSI disability programs, you will also be eligible for medical coverage. Medicare is the medical coverage that comes with SSDI, but its coverage starts two years *after* you are determined eligible to receive your first monthly benefit. Medicaid is the medical coverage that comes with SSI in most states (in California, Medicaid is called MediCal). At the present time, only Medicaid provides reliable payment for medications.

Definition of Disability

At the heart of both disability programs is Social Security's definition of disability. Social Security's concept of disability is difficult to comprehend until you realize that, although they use the word that is found in the English language and is pronounced like the English word "disability," Social Security's use of the term can best be understood as a unique foreign language. Only when you understand this can you work effectively with the definition to your advantage.

Social Security defines *disability* as follows:

". . . The inability to engage in any substantial gainful activity by reason of any medically determinable physical or mental impairment which can be expected to result in death or which has lasted or can be expected to last a continuous period of not less than twelve months."

Do not fight this definition, *but understand it and learn to use it!* Put simply, and in a possibly overstated fashion, what you must prove with your medical evidence to be eligible for disability benefits is that, *if you were hired to do any job* that exists in a *significant number in the national economy, you are unable to do* any *full-time job* in the national economy on a reliable and consistent basis. Whether you have ever done the work, or whether the employer would actually hire you, pay you enough, or that you would want to perform this job is largely irrelevant. In any claim for disability you must address the question of whether you would be *able* to do any kind of work *on a full-time basis,* six to eight hours a day, five days a week. Thus, questions of stamina, reliability, physical/cognitive issues, and ability to handle the reasonable expectations and demands of any employer should clearly be addressed.

As you get older, starting at age fifty, and definitely by age fifty-five, Social Security's assessment of disability will also consider your age as another factor in determining whether you are disabled. Because the decision of whether or not you have "proven" your disability can be made only by the Social Security Administration, a brief written declaration from your doctor declaring that "My patient is totally disabled" is not good enough. However, when that same conclusion is thoroughly documented by your doctor (e.g., your primary care physician or your psychologist), with the medical records that provide a complete history of your doctor's findings and an assessment of your symptoms, then such a letter, with supporting records, could go a long way in ultimately proving your disability, as defined by Social Security.

Information from a certified vocational rehabilitation counselor (CRC) related to your lack of employment potential or to your specific workplace challenges can also be helpful.

Note: Social Security has published a list of impairments with specific clinical findings, which, if medically proven, would entitle you to be found "disabled." (See appendix D-1 for the Listing of Impairments related to MS.)

UNDERSTANDING AND SURVIVING THE APPLICATION/ADMINISTRATIVE PROCESS

When you apply for disability benefits with the Social Security Administration, you can best understand the process you will be engaged in by thinking of it as climbing a ladder. At the top of the ladder are the benefits you seek. It is a very tall ladder with many different rungs, each of which must be used to climb to the top. There is no elevator to the top, and you cannot skip any individual rung. If you are denied at one of the rung levels, as a rule, you should promptly climb to the next rung by appealing that denial rather than dropping your efforts, jumping off the ladder, and starting all over at the bottom. Most importantly, at *every stage* of the administrative process, you normally have only *sixty days to file an appeal* of a prior denial. Do not miss this sixty-day window, because then you will have to start at the bottom rung of the ladder all over again.

Initial Application and Reconsideration

To start your claim for disability benefits with the Social Security Administration, you must file an application. This application process is the first rung of the ladder that must be climbed. *All* applications are made in writing, although frequently you will be asked to provide information over the phone.

After the initial phone interview, a final "hard copy" of that interview will be sent to you to sign and return, along with other papers that might need your signature. These might include release forms so that Social Security can get your medical records. Any additional information you wish to provide is supposed to go through the SSA interviewer who will mail additional information to the Disability Determination Services (DDS) Adjudicator.

In *all* of the numerous forms and papers that you will need to complete and sign, you should be "bluntly and graphically honest" about *all* of the medical, physical, and psychological symptoms that you and/or your friends say "affect" your ability to work. Leaving information out because of personal embarrassment (or modesty) is the easiest way to make sure that the Social Security Administration does not completely assess your claim. We understand that it can be embarrassing for many of you to admit to memory problems, cognitive issues, or bowel/bladder challenges but this is critical information in assessing your ability to work.

It is important for you to make sure that your medical providers and counselors support your claim. If you believe that your MS is so severe that it meets Social Security's standards of disability, but your doctors and counselors do not agree with you, your chances of winning your case will be seriously reduced. Although the Social Security Administration is "supposed" to obtain the records from your medical providers, be aware that it is *your* duty to prove your disability. So, if you can get copies of your doctors' or counselors' records and letters that address your medical limitations and present these to the Social Security Administration, you will then know this information has been obtained and provided to the SSA. Do this as early in the process as possible because it can be difficult to get both clear and appropriate letters within the necessary time frame. Be sure to keep copies of all the papers you gather together and send to Social Security.

Once Social Security has reviewed all the information supplied, they will make a decision known as an *Initial Determination*. You will receive this as a written determination. Usually, this letter doesn't go into great detail about Social Security's analysis of the medical information. Frequently, it is so superficial that it may cause you to become frustrated and angry. If their first decision is a denial, instead of becoming frustrated or angry you should become even more determined.

Within sixty days of the date of the initial determination, you must climb to the next rung of the application ladder by *filing, in writing,* a *Request for Reconsideration* of your denial. All interactions with Social Security should *be in writing, submitted well within the sixty-day deadline.* If you are late, by even one day, Social Security can outright deny your entire claim. *Don't give them this easy out.* You should adopt the reliable strategy of submitting all papers to the Social Security Administration either in person or by certified mail, return receipt requested, and always keeping a copy of every paper submitted in an organized file.

At the reconsideration level, a second look at your case will be made, and you have the right to submit updated medical information. Remember, *always appeal an unfavorable decision well before the expiration of sixty days.*

If a second denial notice is issued, it may be captioned "Notice of Reconsideration." Once again, to protest the unfavorable decision at this level, you should file a protest within sixty days, this time by requesting in writing a *Request for Hearing.*

Administrative Hearing

The next rung to climb of the administrative appeals ladder will be a live, in-person hearing before an administrative law judge. **Note:** Currently, in many hearing offices, Social Security is experiencing delays of *nearly two years* from the time you request a hearing to the date of the actual hearing. Although these hearings are somewhat informal, and no opposing lawyer or jury is present, appearing before any judge can be somewhat intimidating. It is likely that this will be the first time you are face-to-face with the person making the decision in your case. It is not uncommon to find that the judge has called a medical and/or vocational expert to testify and express opinions about your disability.

Also at this hearing, the judge will be applying an enormous set of rules and regulations (about which you will know very little) to your case. The hearing gives you your best opportunity to present in your own words, and possibly brief testimony from your witness, how your medical symptoms prevent you from doing all types of work on a reliable and consistent basis. Although the hearings typically last only for an hour, brief testimony from lay witnesses such as friends or relatives can play a critical role in confirming your limitations. Arranging the live medical testimony of your doctor or another specialist (e.g., your vocational rehabilitation counselor) could be quite helpful, but this can be difficult to arrange due to busy schedules. However, accurate letters from your doctor or counselor can suffice.

An administrative hearing before a Social Security judge might be compared to driving in the Indianapolis 500 car race. The fact that you have a driver's license and have been driving for twenty years doesn't necessarily prepare you to drive in that race. Similarly, the fact that your education and experience have stood you in good stead in your private and professional life doesn't make you a lawyer skilled in the critical nuances of a Social Security disability hearing. Finding and hiring an attorney who has experience representing people like you on a regular basis before Social Security hearings is quite important.

Find an Attorney to Help with Your Social Security Claim

Most experienced lawyers take Social Security cases such as yours on a contingency basis. This means that the lawyer seeks no payment for his or her time unless he or she succeeds at getting you your benefits. Usually, the lawyer's agreement with you will be that he or she is to be paid 25 percent of the retroactive benefits paid to you *only* if you are awarded benefits. All attorney's fees to be charged must be approved by the Social Security Administration, even if both the lawyer and the client have agreed to the fee. If you cannot find a local experienced lawyer to represent you, consider contacting the National Organization of Social Security Claimants' Representatives (NOSSCR). You will find the Web site for NOSSCR listed in the Resources section at the back of the book.

If you haven't consulted a lawyer previously, you should contact a lawyer immediately when you receive a second denial at the "Reconsideration" level. The Social Security Administration maintains a listing of lawyers' organizations who do this type of work—and your local MS organization will also know of attorneys in your area who are familiar with both MS and this process.

Note: *Remember to file your hearing request well within the sixty-day time limit, even if you haven't been able to contact a lawyer.*

Post-Hearing Appeals

In most cases, your judge will not announce his or her decision at the end of your hearing, but will take the case "under advisement," and issue a written decision several weeks to a few months after the hearing. If the judge's decision is unfavorable, further appeals may be taken to the Appeals Council in Falls Church, Virginia, by filing a "Request for Review of Hearing Decision" within sixty days. Unfortunately, delays of more than a year and a half at the Appeals Council are quite common.

Federal Court

If your case is again denied by the Appeals Council, you have sixty days to file a formal appeal in your local federal district court. You should be aware that most lawyers are hesitant to take on new cases for the first time after they have been denied by the Appeals Council because the lawyer has had no input into the preparation or presentation of the case up to that point. Any federal court appeal will be limited to the records presented up to that point. Your best chance to win your case requires the presentation of a comprehensive claim for benefits through a team effort headed by you and supported by your family, friends, healthcare providers, and, at times, your lawyer early in the administrative hearing phase.

When Should You Apply for SSDI/SSI?

The answer to the question posed above is that it really depends on your individual circumstances. As discussed in chapter 8, perhaps you can continue working if your employer can provide you with reasonable accommodations. If you believe that you need to consult with someone about whether your needs can be met by seeking reasonable accommodations, consider discussing your concerns with a neurologist, vocational rehabilitation counselor, or other rehabilitation specialist. Your local state vocational rehabilitation agency or multiple sclerosis organization can also be helpful.

If, however, accommodations were tried and are no longer helpful, or accommodations were not applicable in the first place given your situation, it is probably time to apply for SSDI.

The Social Security Administration has determined that if you are able to earn at least $830 per month (2005 figure), you are not considered disabled by their definition. So, you may ask, "Can I apply (and not be immediately disqualified) for SSDI and still work, as long as I earn less than $830 a month?" The answer to that is a very unreliable "yes," although others may disagree with that. Regardless, you definitely will need to have very strong, accurate, detailed documentation proving that the amount of work you are currently doing is the maximum you can do.

SOME PERSPECTIVES ON THE PROCESS

Sources from which you will need to obtain strong disability documentation include your neurologist or MS specialist, a vocational rehabilitation counselor, or other specialists/professionals with whom you may be working and, hopefully, your employer. Remember, you are claiming that due to your disability(ies), you cannot work at any kind of "full-time" job based on the criteria for "substantial gainful activity."

Swallow Your Pride: Don't Try to Do It All by Yourself

If you don't feel overwhelmed by the application process, then you don't really understand it!

Putting Your Team Together

Your team *must* consist of medical personnel, especially a neurologist and, if applicable, your primary care physician, rehabilitation counselor, neuropsychologist, rehabilitation therapist(s), psychiatrist, and so on. Getting a support letter from your neurologist and other applicable medical people who have treated you recently can be a crucial supplement to your medical records. (See appendix D-2 for sample letters.) Because MS is a disease of the central nervous system, a board-certified neurologist's opinion is given greater weight by the SSA and its courts than an internist's or other medical person's opinion. However, the opinions of your doctors, no matter what their specialties are, must be given great weight by SSA.

Make sure your doctor and therapists have pertinent information in your medical charts because they will be requested by the DDS Adjudicator.

For example, have your telephone conversations with your healthcare providers been entered into your medical chart and if so, do you know what they say? Also, do you know what was added to your chart during your regular office visits? Have you been candid with your doctor about how you are really feeling and functioning: physically, cognitively, and emotionally? If you haven't been candid, begin doing so now. If you have been open and honest about the state of your health, then ask to see your chart to make sure you know what's in it and to make sure the information is accurate.

Note: The support letter from your physician to the Social Security Administration is the most significant. For that reason, make sure that your doctor's letter to the SSA contains all of the information listed in checklist 12 below:

Checklist 12: Your Physician's Letter

_____ His or her accreditations and/or credentials and signature appear on any correspondence to the SSA

_____ What your formal diagnosis is and the date of your diagnosis

_____ When your symptoms started to occur

_____ How MS limits your activities and how it would limit work-related activities (provide the doctor with a description of your job and check off the job tasks or functions that are limited by your MS). It can also be helpful if your spouse (or significant other) and your vocational rehabilitation counselor write a letter on your behalf noting observations they have made about your limitations. That is, they can check off tasks or functions that are difficult or impossible for you to perform. This would include both daily activities like dressing and housekeeping, and work activities like typing, planning, remembering, organizing, and so forth. It is important for your doctor to refer in the support letter to how each of these types of activities is compromised because of your disabled condition.

_____ What your medical tests have shown

_____ What treatment(s) you have received including what worked and what didn't work

_____ Your likely medical future (this information is of critical importance to the SSA)

Cognitive and Emotional Issues

If your symptoms include cognitive and/or emotional issues, and you have seen a neuropsychologist and/or a psychotherapist or other type of practitioner for these problems, having that practitioner write a support letter for you can be very helpful. Most people with MS have stopped working more because of their cognitive problems than because of their physical or emotional issues. Allow us to repeat ourselves: We know that it can be hard to be honest about (or even to understand) lapses in memory and problem-solving skills, or other issues involved in thinking clearly. But this is not your job. This is the role of the neuropsychologist.

A support letter from the neuropsychologist who did your neuropsychological evaluation can be critical. Ideally, the letter needs to include the elements listed above along with a summary of the results from the testing (a four- to eight-hour battery of tests) and what conclusions can be made in terms of your ability to work at substantial gainful activity. (See chapter 10 for a complete discussion of neuropsychological testing.) Likewise, if you have been seeing a psychotherapist, a support letter from him or her can also be helpful and should include the elements listed in the checklist above. Often, your neuropsychologist can also address your emotional issues.

Former Employers

Sometimes, your former employer(s) will be willing to write a support letter on your behalf. He or she can attest to the functioning problems you were having that affected your ability to work. This can range from attendance and dependability issues to productivity and quality of work. Needless to say, this may be the only time when information about your getting fired, laid off, or having resigned from a job can actually help you. If a former employer is not willing to write a letter or you're not comfortable asking him or her to do so, attach a copy of your job performance evaluations that indicate problems and explain how these problems were caused by or related to your various symptoms. Some truly supportive employers may actually be good witnesses for you at a hearing.

Emotional Support

Okay. Touchy-feely can be good. It can be very helpful to secure everyday emotional support and assistance. But, it can be absolutely critical in helping you through the very personal and difficult Social Security application process for a variety of reasons. One such reason is that during this application process you will need to acknowledge the many losses you've suffered due to the MS and how it has impacted not only your ability to work, but your entire life. It can also be helpful if your psychotherapist, significant other, or friends write a letter for you documenting the emotional stresses you are experiencing.

Hands-on Assistance

Lastly, if available, an MS social worker or counselor knowledgeable about the process of applying for SSDI and SSI and what the Disability Determination Services Adjudicator looks for in answers to the application questions can be instrumental in helping you to win your claim. You may receive an offer from the Social Security intake person or from an SSI facilitator to help you fill out the application form. Thank them for their offer, but do it yourself with your own advocate or team. You and your team have far more incentive to do a comprehensive and well-written application than a Social Security Administration employee or state employee.

Applying for SSDI Is Your Full-time Job

You have now embarked on a real, frustrating, demanding, and time-consuming process. Expect to spend eight to twelve hours minimum engaged in the following tasks:

- setting up your team,

- coordinating their separate pieces of documentation,

- gathering pertinent information,

- doing the prep work,

- drafting comprehensive and concise answers to the questions on the application form,

- reviewing your answers until you and your team are satisfied,

- writing a cover letter stating what attachments you are including,

- making copies of everything you plan to send to SSA by certified mail (or bring to the SSA interview), and then

- sending it.

Note: An experienced MS advocate should review all of your responses to application form questions before you give your application form to the SSA.

Prepare Yourself Mentally for This Endeavor

This is not the time to make the best of a bad situation. For the next few weeks, filing for SSDI will be your "job." Do not pretty things up. It is crucial that you be honest, objective, and forthcoming about the severity of the symptoms that cause your inability to work at substantial gainful activity (SGA). This means *all* of your applicable symptoms including very personal and perhaps embarrassing ones. This is not a time to tone down what is really going on. Be blunt and graphically honest about the full range of your symptoms and limitations.

Prepare Emotionally for Saying What You Need to Say

Think of the well-known Native American saying: "Walk a while in my moccasins before you judge me." You want the person who will review your application to be able to walk in your shoes twenty-four hours a day, seven days a week, based on the information you provide. Your objective is to separate you, the unique individual, from the you who is the applicant who deserves these benefits. The challenge to you and your supporters is for you to become one of the 30 to 35 percent of applicants who win their claim the first time around.

To do this, you must be honest with yourself and acknowledge all the symptoms that have a negative impact on your daily activities and your ability to work. You must also be willing to accept what people close to you have observed about any cognitive impairment you have demonstrated, as an example, and include this in your application. This type of impairment can be documented in letters from several of your friends. If their observations can be medically or psychologically documented, then you would want to include this documentation in the appropriate section on the form. Again, this is not the time to put your best face forward. Be completely truthful about all of the limitations you've had to endure.

HOT TIPS ABSTRACTED FROM THE SSDI TUTOR*

by Rebecca Pursely

Do Your Homework

Before contacting Social Security, you should gather all of the necessary information you will need to fill out the application form and get a strong rough draft completed. Once you have done this, then contact Social Security and officially begin the process. Once you contact them and get into the system, the clock starts ticking for when you must have it all turned in. Although they won't tell you this, you actually have six months to complete the application process. Naturally, however, you don't want to wait that long. On the other hand, you don't want to feel the pressure and stress of being given an arbitrary deadline by the Social Security people.

McKee's Twelve Rules for Dealing with Bureaucracies

1. **Get and stay organized.** Do not rely on Social Security (or any other bureaucracy) to keep track of your papers, phone calls, and other contacts with them. Assume that they will lose things and you will have to prove that you filed critical papers on time. Keep copies of every paper you sign or give to Social Security. If mailing any papers to Social Security, send them by certified mail, return receipt requested, and staple the return card to your copy, which you keep in a chronological file.

2. **Name and number.** Whenever you talk to someone by phone, do not hang up until you have his or her name, address, direct telephone number, and if need be, his or her fax number.

3. **Says who?** When given an answer you think is wrong, confused (or you just don't like), politely ask for a copy of the written authority which is said to explain/justify/require the person's answer.

4. **Official policy ploy.** If the ultimate fallback position of the person you are talking to is that "official policy/office policy" is the basis of their answer, express your doubt about this answer, and ask to see a written copy of that policy.

5. **Call the boss.** For almost every person you speak to in a bureaucracy, that person has a boss or supervisor who may have a completely different (and possibly more favorable) answer to your request. Talk to that supervisor/boss. Keep climbing the ladder. When all else fails, if your claim is getting no action and has become "stuck" or "lost," consider contacting your local congressional representative. A congressional inquiry sometimes can "shake things loose," but it *cannot* affect Social Security's ultimate decision as to whether you are disabled.

---

* Acknowledgment—We thank Rebecca for the gracious use of her currently unpublished *The SSDI Tutor*, her participation as copresenter of the materials from her Multiple Sclerosis Association of King County's SSDI/SSI workshops over the past several years, and for her perseverance and dedication to helping others with their applications in spite of "bad days" with her MS.

6. **Document, document, document.** Assume that if it isn't confirmed by writing, and it isn't in your hand, then it doesn't exist. This applies to anything that people say has happened, say is going to happen, and to things that you say you have done.

7. **No snow job.** When someone gives you an answer to your question or request, don't say, "Yes, I understand," when you're really thinking "What the heck does *that* mean?" Make that person explain it down or up to your level. Work through the anger you may feel and persevere.

8. **Set a deadline.** When someone says he or she will get back to you with answers to your request, set a definite date for that to happen (at least in your own mind). When that date arrives, almost regardless of what has subsequently taken place, write *one* follow-up request, and then, if you don't receive a reply in a short period of time, assume that person will *not* do what he or she promised, and plan another strategy.

9. **Don't quit.** Be persistent. The main defense a bureaucracy has is its great ability to out-wait those who request it to take actions. Take a perverse pride in your ability to demonstrate greater stamina and tenacity than the bureaucracy personnel.

10. **Know when to quit.** There are times when you must drop your long-pursued approach to achieving your goals. It's okay to be determined, but it's not okay to become obsessed.

11. **Know the pros.** Maintain a list of names and phone numbers of the people in the bureaucracies with whom you deal who really know their stuff, have shown themselves to be caring and willing to do what they promise, and have a record of actually getting the job done. Be nice to these people, above all others.

12. **Be professional.** At all times, be professional, courteous, and honest. Your credibility in the entire application process is the key element to your disability claim.

Start a daily journal NOW! This can actually be used as documentation. Items to be documented include such things as the following:

- An outline of your activities on an ordinary day. Appendix D-3, the Daily Activity Questionnaire, can be helpful to review here.

- The location, duration, frequency, and intensity of your pain or other symptoms.

- The factors that trigger or worsen your pain or other symptoms.

- The type, dosage, effectiveness, and side effects of any medication.

- Treatments, other than medications, that you take for your pain and other symptoms.

- Name your worst/most troublesome symptom, then rate it on a nuisance scale from 1 to 10 each day. It can be helpful to utilize the rating scales you will find in appendix D-4.

- Keep a calendar by your bed and write "good," "bad," or "okay" on the date before you nod off to sleep.

Sample Journal Page			Day/Date:
Time	Activities	Pain Triggers	Pain Location, Duration, Frequency and Intensity (0–10) of Discomfort
7–8 A.M.			
8–9 A.M.			
9–10 A.M.			
10–11 A.M.			
11 A.M.–12 P.M.			
and so on . . .			
Medications and side effects:			
Other treatment:			
Most troublesome symptom(s):			Rating 0–10 as to discomfort

Keep Records of Everything Related to Your Health and Disability

Phone calls. Record the (1) date and time of call, (2) the names of people you talked to, with (3) their titles, (4) affiliations, (5) phone numbers, and (6) conversation highlights. See the form below for a sample of how to document a phone call:

_____

Sample Phone Call Documentation

Date and Time: _____   Conversation with: _____

Title of person you're calling: _____

Summary of Conversation: _____

_____

_____

_____

Dates. Write the name of the item and the dates that you requested the item, received it, sent or delivered it, and followed up with a phone call, letter, or visit.

Letters, notices, and forms. *Keep all correspondence.* Register all mail correspondence you send to SSA or the DDS Adjudicator and write "return receipt requested" on the front of the envelope. Get receipts for all items you deliver personally.

Make two copies of all documents you send to SSA/DDS. Submit the original but keep two copies. One copy is for your reference so that you don't contradict yourself if SSA/DDS requests more information. It can also be useful if you need to fill out any other type of insurance forms. The second copy is a spare in case your original disappears.

Prepare to wait. When you call SSA, expect to be on hold for annoyingly long periods of time, especially if you are calling the local office as opposed to the 800-772-1213 number. Anticipate a wait and plan something to do while you wait. If you visit a Social Security office, bring any medications you may need to take over the next three to four hours. Once you've submitted your application form, you will most likely be asked to submit additional information to complete your application. Once these forms have been turned in, it's always a good idea to check back in a couple of weeks to make sure DDS received all the requested documentation and be sure to ask if there is anything else they need. After you have confirmed this, expect to wait two to three months for a decision.

THE NITTY-GRITTY: THE NARRATIVE SECTIONS

There are at least five questions SSA routinely asks for which you will need more room than the tiny spaces provided by the application form. These questions are as follows:

- An in-depth description of *what* your multiple sclerosis symptoms are and *how* they affect you.

- A detailed assessment of *how* your MS symptoms limit your ability to work at any type of job.

- A complete list of the job-related changes you had to make because of your multiple sclerosis.

- The specific reasons why you stopped working.

- A comprehensive review of the job you held the longest and the duties you performed.

This last question probably won't be a problem to answer, although you can approach your answer by breaking down your job duties and responsibilities into three parts: the thinking part of your job (cognitive), the physical demands part of your job, and the emotional/psychological aspects of your job. The latter refers to the job stresses, such as supervising and/or interactions with coworkers, managers, or customers, deadlines, financial responsibilities, safety responsibilities, and so forth.

The first four bulleted items are a different matter. It is **very** important for you to be *thorough, comprehensive,* and *concise* in your answers. The following pages will help you by describing useful writing techniques and organizational strategies to employ. As Ms. Pursely says, "Yes, this is a *major* undertaking.

Yes, it is a pain. Yes, you shouldn't have to go through all this to get your own money. Yes, it stinks. And, yes, it's necessary."

Suggestions and Examples

Whenever possible, go for answers that create a clear picture of the point you're trying to make. Try to illustrate your point with comparisons or contrasts:

- *Example:* A year ago I averaged eight hours of sleep a night and took a daily half-hour nap. Currently, I need ten hours of sleep each night and I require a half-hour nap in the morning and an hour nap in the afternoon to be able to complete my day.

- *Example:* One year ago, I did all the shopping (twice a week), prepared dinners, and did the laundry and cleaning. Six months ago, I had to reduce this to shopping once a week, cooking every other dinner, no laundry, and cleaning only the bathrooms and kitchen. Today, I fix one dinner a week, and help only marginally with cleaning the kitchen. These changes have occurred because of my fatigue, pain, and balance problems.

You may also want to use "if/then" or "else" or "cause and effect" statements:

- *Example:* If I walk briskly for more than ten strides, then my legs become too weak to support my body.

- *Example:* I must hold on to the grocery cart at the store or else I fall into the shelves.

- *Example:* Riding in a car for longer than fifteen minutes causes my legs to go numb.

Organizing Your Narrative Answers

To help you frame your answers, see appendix D-4 for diary-format and applicable worksheets. Remember, the disability application form is for anyone who claims he or she is unable to work due to his or her disability or disabilities. As Rebecca Pursely says, "The challenge is to state your case adequately within a form that's better suited to a disease or condition with a single symptom." In other words, not multiple sclerosis.

There are four worksheets included in appendix D-4. Because fatigue is a major MS symptom, there are two worksheets especially for fatigue. The other two worksheets can be used to describe your other symptoms.

Note: There are four steps to filling out these worksheets:

1. Make a list of *ALL* of your symptoms. If you have more than one disease or condition, include those symptoms as well. Remember: *you* are applying, not your MS.

2. Make a copy of the worksheets in appendix D-4 for *each* symptom you have.

3. Complete the worksheets.

4. Use the information from page 1 of each worksheet to answer the questions on the application under Part 1 4A, where they ask you to describe your condition. Use the information from page 2 of each worksheet to answer the questions on the application under Part 1 4B and 5, where they ask you to describe your symptoms that affect basic work actitivies.

Cognitive and Emotional Symptoms

Leading experts in the field put the percentage of people with MS who do or will experience cognitive problems during their lifetime as a majority. Also, experts in the field indicate that the percentage of those with MS who do now or will experience depression in the future is extremely high, as are mood swings. What this means is that cognitive and emotional issues are not something you can ignore or should keep secret when applying for SSDI or SSI.

It may well be the case that a majority of claimants for Social Security disability benefits were forced to stop work because of their cognitive problems. If cognitive and/or emotional problems are part of the reason you are applying for either SSDI or SSI *and you state this on the application form,* expect to receive a notice from either the DDS or SSA that they will need to schedule you for an assessment with a psychologist.

They will send you to someone who has agreed to accept the amount of money the SSA will pay. Will that person have any experience with MS? It's doubtful. Will that person play a role in determining your fate? Absolutely! Therefore, when you receive notice from the DDS Adjudicator, call back, make the appointment, and, if cognitive impairments are your issue, be sure to send a written request for a full neuropsychological evaluation. They won't pay for a full battery of tests but they may well pay for a mini-neuropsychological evaluation. Even if they refuse your request and set you up for the traditional fifty-minute session, at least you will have documentation of what you requested. (Remember, you must keep two copies of everything you send to them.)

This may be helpful if you are denied benefits, and you appeal the decision. Ideally, you will already have had a full neuropsychological evaluation done by someone of your choosing via a referral from your neurologist/team, or you will already be seeing a psychologist or psychotherapist for emotional issues. Usually, but not always, a report by those treating you will satisfy the reviewer of your claim.

Conclusion

You have worked very hard over the course of your career and you were told that the money you put into Social Security was an insurance plan (financial benefit) for either the day you retire on your own terms or for the day you retire due to a disability. Unfortunately, too often the Social Security process for disability benefits has become an adversarial process. It is Goliath and you are David. Therefore, you need a team comprised of people who are informed, willing to help, emotionally supportive, and capable of assisting you through this arduous process called "Applying for Social Security Disability Benefits." You can triumph, but you must be very persistent and well-organized. Our very best wishes to you during this difficult process.

CHAPTER 12

The Caring Experience: Developing a Partnership

Estelle R. Klasner, Ph.D., Kathryn M. Yorkston, Ph.D., BC-NCD, and Kurt L. Johnson, Ph.D., C.R.C.

A PERSPECTIVE ON CARE AND CAREGIVING

The term "care" has a number of different meanings. Care can mean that you pay special attention to something of value (e.g., "I'm going to take care when I finish this important project"). It can mean to have a high regard for something or someone (e.g., "I truly care for my husband"). "Care" can also mean a worry or responsibility (e.g., "He is troubled by the many cares in his life"). At one time or another, all of these different meanings may describe your thoughts about multiple sclerosis (MS). Multiple sclerosis is a progressive disease, meaning that, over time, it can worsen. You may reach a stage in your disease when you will need other people to care for you. Both needing and giving care are complex roles filled with a whole host of emotions. Providing care may be stressful and frustrating, but it also can present opportunities to discover hidden strengths and feel new joys.

Usually, being someone who requires care or becoming a care provider are not roles that people choose on their own. As a rule, the need for a care provider comes about when someone has a chronic illness, like MS, that interferes with that person's ability to perform activities and tasks independently, on a daily basis. This chapter's purpose is to provide an overview of the issues that must be considered as you begin to establish and maintain a caring partnership between yourself and the family members and/or friends who are helping you. This chapter offers advice to the person with the illness who needs care and the family members and friends who provide care. The term "family," as it is used here, distinguishes between caregivers who are family members and/or friends and those individuals who are paid to give care.

FAMILY CAREGIVERS: WHO YOU ARE AND WHAT YOU DO

Family caregivers are men and women who assist loved ones who have MS. Most often, they are spouses, but they also can be children, parents, or friends. The family caregiver usually assists the person with MS in his or her own home and community, so that the person can maintain a familiar, safe, and secure environment. If you are a family caregiver, you might be involved in a number of activities with the person who has MS. You may assist with shopping, making appointments, driving, and household maintenance. You may also provide companionship and encouragement on a continual basis.

As time goes on, you may be asked to help with such matters as bathing, dressing, and feeding. Your role is very important. You may be the reason a young mother can continue to care for her children, or the reason someone with MS is able to remain in his or her own home. Providing care and support in a kind and compassionate manner, although certainly challenging, can be a rewarding experience.

Recently, the term "caregiver" has come under scrutiny in both the professional and popular press. Some professionals in the field of chronic illness, particularly in Great Britain, have stated that the term implies a one-way relationship, i.e., that the person with MS is getting care and not playing an active role in the relationship. For this reason, the term "carer" has become popular in European countries. In the U.S., the term "care partner" is becoming widely used to refer to both the person with MS and the person giving care. The term "care partner" implies just that, a partnership between two people in which both partners make a contribution. We hope that the information in this chapter will be helpful to you, as you establish your own caring partnership.

THE SPECIAL CASE OF MS

Multiple sclerosis is a disease with some unique characteristics that can have an influence on the caring partnership. First, it is important to note that MS affects more women than men. Because of this, men are more likely to take on the role of the care partner who provides assistance. Traditionally, men have not often taken on caring responsibilities. Research has shown that men approach the caring partnership differently than women (Good, Bower, and Einsporn 1995). Men are less likely to ask for outside help, and they are reluctant to express their feelings about the caring situation. Problems may arise because of the lack of communication and/or insufficient help.

Fortunately, there are solutions for these problems. For example, it should be possible to structure communication situations so that the male caregiver can begin to feel more comfortable sharing his thoughts and feelings. This may require the female care partner to initiate such discussions fairly often.

In another example, outside help may be arranged so that others who are familiar with caring demands can assist. Women are accustomed to assuming a caring role more often than men. However, they are also less likely to take breaks from the care situation, and they often neglect their own health. Becoming aware of the types of issues that may arise allows care partners to set up contingency plans before problems become acute.

Women who provide care might schedule some time each day to take part in health-promoting activities for themselves, like exercise. And they should schedule regular doctor's appointments to monitor their own health. They can also prearrange respite care, so that they will be more inclined to take breaks for rest and relaxation for themselves.

Because MS is a disease that primarily occurs between the ages of twenty to forty years, children or parents can also be care partners. Asking children to take on care responsibilities needs to be carefully considered. Tasks should be appropriate for the age of the child. Certainly, children can contribute to household maintenance, but asking a child to give medications or to carry out personal care tasks such as toileting may be ill-advised. It is very hard to preserve the parent-child relationship when children and parents do not maintain preestablished boundaries.

Most likely children will be eager to help, but parents should clearly delineate the limits of the care they accept from their children. Often, the parents of adult children also act as care partners in many situations. Although this may seem like a natural role for the parent to assume in this situation, caution should be taken to avoid burdening an aging parent. Also, parents need to remember that their "child" is now an adult and should be treated accordingly. It may be wise to have a discussion about "parent-child" roles to avoid the pitfalls that can occur.

Two of the hallmark features of MS are the unpredictability of symptoms and the course the disease takes. Some of you have described having MS and caring for a person with MS as similar to walking on sand; everything shifts and changes all the time. The unpredictable nature of MS makes it essential for care partners to be flexible and able to adapt to changing needs.

For example, you may be able to walk to the mailbox one day, but on the next day, you may only be able to sit on the front porch. This means that care partners must take and give back responsibilities for tasks on a consistent basis. Care partners need to develop an understanding that allows both of the people in the relationship to give and receive the assistance they need.

THE JOURNEY OF CARING

A care partnership cannot be created overnight. It is a dynamic process, and like most other relationships it goes through a series of stages. A number of researchers have investigated the caring partnership and have recognized a series of steps that generally take place. One group of researchers (McKeon and Porter-Armstrong 2004) has defined these steps as *rejecting care, resisting care, seeking care,* and *accepting care.* Both care partners can be engaged in a number of these steps.

Rejecting care. Care is usually rejected at the beginning of the caring partnership. At this stage, both of you as partners refuse outside offers of help in order to maintain independence, protect each other from the changes that MS may bring, and preserve the family as it was before MS.

Resisting care. The next step, resisting care, happens when the care partner without MS acknowledges that he or she may need help but is reluctant to ask for it. He or she gradually takes on more responsibilities and this becomes the "norm." Many care partners, especially spouses, feel that they should be doing all of the care all of the time, and asking for help is not an acceptable option. Neither of you wants to be viewed by others as unable to cope, and asking for help may signify an inability to cope for some people.

Seeking care. Often, the next step in the caring partnership is to seek care. Frequently, this occurs during a period of crisis when you, the person with MS, may be experiencing both an exacerbation and a change in your ability to be independent. At this phase, outside or paid help on a temporary basis is usually sought.

Accepting care. Often, accepting care is the last step for care partners. Both care partners acknowledge that the situation has evolved to the point where it is necessary to obtain additional help. Care partners may increase their reliance on other family members or they may make a more permanent arrangement with paid-care providers.

Being aware of the stages that a caring partnership may undergo allows both partners to practice patience and realize that their partnership will change and shift in sympathy with the care needs of both partners.

CARE PARTNERSHIP BASICS: FIRST THINGS FIRST

Even when a spouse or other close relative has provided care for someone he or she has lived with for a number of years, the establishment of a caring partnership in the face of MS is a new venture. Some issues must be addressed early on to ensure a successful partnership. Becoming educated about MS, deciding on a primary care partner, and establishing house rules are some of the basics that need to be put in place at the start of the partnership and they should continue to be monitored throughout the care process.

Become Educated About MS

Research suggests that caregivers who view themselves as prepared and knowledgeable about the disability experience less strain than those who feel less prepared (McKeon and Porter-Armstrong 2004). It is important for care partners to first gain a full understanding of MS and all of the symptoms that may occur. Information is available from a number of resources including your doctor, nurse, books, and the Internet. Becoming aware of all of the aspects of MS that may occur can help you, as care partners, to develop plans for care and goals that are logical and realistic. Also, you may wish to share this information with your family and friends, so that if a situation arises in which that friend or family member is to provide care, he or she will know what to expect.

New developments in the treatment of MS are occurring at a rapid rate. It is necessary to keep abreast of these developments and discuss them with your healthcare provider(s) to determine whether the new treatment might be appropriate for the person with MS. Chapter 1, Optimizing Your Medical Management, and chapter 6, Alternative Therapy Considerations, are excellent places to start educating yourself about MS.

Decide on a Primary Care Partner

One person should be chosen as the primary care partner. The primary care partner is the person who is responsible for organizing all of the care that is needed. As a primary care partner, you work out schedules with the person who has MS and you communicate with all of the other care partners. In addition, the primary care partner knows all of the important medical information such as doctor's name, allergies, and medication schedule. He or she also knows where things are stored and how the home is organized. As the disease progresses, the primary care partner also may have to become aware of new medical and daily routines. The primary care partner and the person with MS make all major decisions and plans for the inevitable changes that occur as a result of MS.

Establishing a primary care partner is a good way to avoid poor communication. One person acting as the primary resource allows the other caregivers to know how and where to access important information. It also allows other caregivers to feel confident that the care they provide was designed in conjunction with the person who has MS. If and when problems arise, the other caregivers can be assured that decisions will be made by the primary care partner and the person with MS.

Establish House Rules

Most people have particular ways they like things done in their own home and ways they prefer to be approached and treated. It is essential for care partners to establish rules early on in the caring partnership. Rules regarding personal care and household tasks should be decided on from the outset of the partnership. For example, care partners may decide that only the primary care partner should administer medication. Housecleaning, cooking, and pet care may be other areas in which rules need to be set. Care partners also must decide about daily routines such as times for meals, exercise, treatment, and bedtimes.

If children are living in the home, schedules are of the utmost importance. Having an organized daily routine will ensure allowing enough time to help children with their schoolwork and any other tasks they need to perform. This type of organization allows for care partners to take on as many duties as they wish to, while capitalizing on each other's strengths and being aware of each other's limitations. It also provides an opportunity for care partners to discuss expectations and remain realistic about what can be accomplished. See chapter 2, Getting Things Done: Managing Your Time and Energy, for details about planning and carrying out preferred activities.

DIFFERENT VIEWS: CARE PARTNER PERSPECTIVES

Each care partner comes to the relationship with his or her own set of personal qualities and experiences. These distinctive qualities often add richness and a unique level of understanding that is vital for a successful caring partnership. To benefit from each other's differences, these differences must be recognized and respected by each of you. In addition, the complex nature of your partnership must be acknowledged, and care partners need to recognize that the partnership will go through "good" and "bad" times. Care partners should acknowledge differing viewpoints, the potential for both positive and negative feelings, and the time required to adjust to the changes brought about by MS.

Recognizing Your Care Partner Differences

Care partners will inevitably have different views on a number of issues. If you have MS, you see the care partner relationship from "inside" the disease. You must make constant adjustments to your new role and be willing to accept care. You must also come to terms with the changing roles that MS has imposed on you. For example, a husband who was the sole breadwinner may now have to share this responsibility with his wife and he may need to spend more time on tasks at home such as helping children with homework and preparing meals.

When you are the primary care partner, you must view the partnership from "outside" of the disease. A care partner may have to assume a number of extra responsibilities. He or she may have to adjust work schedules and take on more household tasks.

The different perspectives you have as care partners can create different priorities for each person. If you are the person with MS, at times, you may want your care partner to be available at all times, and or you may feel resentment toward the person without MS. If you are the care partner providing care, you may also feel resentment about life adjustments, decreased financial security, and increased responsibilities. Both of you care partners need to "take stock" on a regular basis and monitor both sets of needs and expectations. You need to ask yourselves if demands are reasonable, and acknowledge the challenge of each other's position in the caring partnership.

Feelings: Positive and Negative

A caring partnership is filled with emotion. Often, spouses, children, parents, relatives, and friends are kind, compassionate care partners, and are invaluable resources. However, dealing with MS on a daily basis can be difficult. Adjustments to role shifts, loss of intimacy, loss of privacy, an increased sense of vulnerability, and living with uncertainty are often necessary. These changes will frequently cause feelings of resentment, anger, and jealousy.

At the same time, care partners may discover hidden strengths and resources. You may also find new activities to share. Whether positive or negative, emotions should be discussed in an open manner if that is at all possible. One way to facilitate conversations about challenging issues is to set aside a time for discussion. It is nearly impossible to come to any resolution if discussions take place during a trying or difficult situation. Emotions are generally high and care partners need time away from the situation to decide on a reasonable and realistic plan for dealing with difficult matters. It may be necessary to seek outside professional help such as a counselor, religious advisor, or mental health professional to help you, as care partners, to talk about your problems. Seeking outside help should be done sooner, rather than later, to avoid escalation of negative emotions, which if left unchecked, can turn into abusive situations.

Care Partners Need Time to Adjust

If you have MS, you also may have ongoing, ever-changing emotions about having the disease. You must deal with the knowledge of having a progressive illness and that this illness will be a major influence on your plans for your life. Because of the changes that MS causes, those having the disease must cope with loss of function and possibly loss of control over certain situations on an ongoing basis.

If you are the primary care partner, you must also deal with change and loss. You may need to work outside the home and give up staying at home during the day to care for the children. You, too, may have to change your life plans because of MS. For example, you may have to choose to turn down a promotion because the new position entails a great deal of traveling. You may have a hard time juggling care responsibilities, work, and children. Care partners may have to learn how and when to ask for help. You may require time to adjust to your new life situations. Respect between care partners for each other's situation is one of the most helpful ways to cope with adjustment issues and to prepare for the future.

GIVE AND TAKE: THE NEEDS OF CARE PARTNERS

Throughout this chapter, we have emphasized the "partnership" involved in caring for a family member with MS. It is critical that both partners be cared for. While care partners are busy with the duties involved in the caring partnership, it must be remembered that you both have individual needs. Both of you need time to care for yourselves. And both of you will benefit from time away from each other to pursue other activities and interests that have nothing to do with your roles as care partners. Maintaining social and leisure interests is essential to staying balanced and content in any partnership.

Taking Care of Yourself

Maintaining a sense of well-being is one of the most important things that care partners can do for each other. Care partners must strive to keep a healthy balance between the physical, emotional, and social aspects of life. Because much of this book focuses on the person with MS, this chapter will emphasize the need for a primary care partner to take care of him- or herself. For the primary care partner, physical well-being involves eating a nutritious diet, exercising whenever possible, getting enough rest, and tending to personal medical needs. When providing assistance, primary care partners often neglect their own needs and do not receive necessary medical attention. One of the greatest gifts that you can give to your family member with MS is taking care of yourself on a regular basis.

Maintaining your emotional well-being can be a juggling act. At times, both care partners are bound to feel depressed, angry, and anxious. However, it's important for care partners to recognize when these negative feelings may become problematic, that is, it's important to recognize when these feelings may pose a problem. For example, care partners may experience depression that goes unrecognized. (See chapter 5 for a discussion of ways to deal with depression and other emotional challenges.)

It's also important for care partners to maintain their social well-being. Care partners often feel trapped and isolated in their situation. Becoming isolated can happen so gradually that both care partners may not be aware of the situation for some time. Maintaining social connections is vital to a balanced partnership. Both care partners should continue to engage in activities they have always enjoyed, separately and together.

If going out is difficult, having an occasional potluck dinner may provide much needed social interaction. Friends can gather at one care partner's home and bring dinner with them so that neither care partner is burdened with transportation or cooking duties. Other social activities might include listening to music, renting movies, playing cards or board games, visiting art galleries, museums, or libraries, if possible, and learning something new like a foreign language or new computer program.

Respite Is Both Needed and Necessary

Both care partners will benefit from frequent and regularly scheduled respite from each other. Time away creates a sense of security for both care partners. You, having the disability, acknowledge that other people can provide competent care. Your primary care partner acknowledges that it is possible to delegate his or her caring responsibilities to other people. You may need a break from your primary care partner often in order to feel confident that you can get along with someone else's help and spend time with others. This allows you to maintain a social network with previous friends and relatives.

Obviously, the primary care partner also benefits from regularly scheduled respite. Primary care partners often report experiencing social isolation due to fatigue resulting from the demands of taking care of someone else and decreased interaction with others.

Respite also allows the care partner to take care of his or her own health issues and spend leisure time with family members or friends. Respite lets the primary caregiver enjoy some unscheduled time that allows him or her to "recharge" his or her energy. When both care partners take some time away from each other, that permits them to engage in a period of reflection and then they may both be able to bring new ideas back to each other for solving difficult situations.

Arranging alternative care should be done in advance and both care partners must be comfortable with the alternative care plans. If family members or friends are not available to provide respite care, services in your community are likely available. Check with your physician or local healthcare center about respite services in your area.

A Word About Paid Respite/Care Help

Although this chapter was written for family caregivers and their loved ones, there may be times when paid-care help is needed. Once the decision has been made to hire someone to assist with care, care partners should consider the available choices very carefully. The level of outside help needed should be discussed.

Several levels of paid help are available, including domestic help, personal care assistants, therapists, certified nursing assistants, and registered nurses. Both care partners should decide which type of care is needed so that an appropriate person can be hired. Care partners also need to discuss financial and privacy issues as they relate to the paid-care provider. Expectations relative to paid assistance should be clear for both care partners.

Finding Paid-Care Help

Going through a licensed agency is one way to hire paid help. Agencies handle all the bookkeeping duties and they are responsible for screening potential employees. Agencies also have the capacity to provide backup care if someone falls ill or care is needed in an emergency. However, agencies also control how many hours care providers can work and the tasks they do. Hiring someone without going through an agency allows for greater control over wages and duties, and may be less costly, as long as there is a reasonable quality of performance.

Churches, synagogues, and other religious facilities may be able to find reliable personnel at modest hourly rates. It is unlikely, however, that religious facilities will conduct background checks or take care of accounting tasks. These will become new responsibilities for both care partners in the event that paid-care help is obtained through religious or community facilities. Moreover, if someone is ill or an emergency arises, substitute care providers will not be available.

In addition to discussing where to hire help and the type of help that is needed, care partners also may want to revisit their house rules and make some changes to feel comfortable with paid help in their home. When your home is open to others on a consistent basis, private information may be inadvertently left out in the open. For example, you both may decide to keep important documents or valuable possessions in a safe-deposit box or fireproof safe in the home to ensure your desired level of privacy. The best way to establish and maintain the desired level of privacy is to take the necessary steps to ensure that privacy. This can go a long way in avoiding embarrassment and unpleasantness between care partners and paid-care helpers.

Informal Support Networks

Family members and friends are often invaluable resources to support care partners. If possible, friends and family can be relied on to help with household projects, running errands, pleasure outings where extra help may be needed, or caring for others in the household, such as children. In addition, care partners often discover that an informal support system already exists in their neighborhood that was formed by everyday contact with members of their community. Frequently, care partners engage in ongoing interactions with postal workers, pharmacists, grocery clerks, neighbors, and other people in their neighborhood.

As time passes, service providers in the neighborhood become aware of the needs of the care partners and can provide support and assistance in recurring situations. For example, a pharmacist may know that because of your disability, you need to sit down while signing for your prescription, and he or she will have a chair available for you. The postal worker may knock on your door and personally deliver packages to you because he or she knows about the difficulty you experience when navigating your way to the mailbox. The grocery store clerk may keep certain items in stock to ensure they are available because you buy them on a regular basis.

Many people in your community will often be interested in providing assistance in any way they can, so that you, as someone with a disability, can continue to live in your own home and neighborhood. These small measures can go a long way to making life easier for care partners. Members of your community often provide more direct support. Some communities have established "telephone trees" to support those with severe disabilities who live in those communities.

For example, if you live at home on your own, neighbors can organize a schedule of calling you periodically to check in and find out if you need any assistance. Telephone trees of support have worked miracles in providing reassurance to care partners. You, as someone with MS, can rest assured that there are people available to provide help, if needed, and the well care partner can go to work or do errands with the confidence of knowing that help will be provided if it becomes necessary. Please remember that it is okay to ask for this help in different life areas.

Maintaining Your Previous Relationship

Often, primary care partners become so focused on the caring routines that they forget they were in another kind of primary relationship with the person with the disability, e.g., husband and wife or parent and adult child. This prior relationship inevitably will weather some changes while the care partnership becomes firmly established. Being able to delegate tasks to others like housecleaning or yard work, on a regular or even occasional basis, will free up time to spend nurturing loving relationships and sharing enjoyable activities.

Activities may involve taking a break from the routine and devoting some time to pleasurable outings such as going to a movie, visiting friends, or taking a scenic drive. This time away from home will provide a much-needed break for you as care partners and also help you to maintain your previously established relationships. You may not be able to engage in pleasurable activities with the same degree of spontaneity that you once enjoyed, but with careful planning both care partners certainly can enjoy leisure time together.

MAKING THE REWARDS OUTWEIGH THE WORRIES: A SET OF GUIDED EXERCISES

At this point, some general issues related to developing a care partnership to deal with MS have been identified. We've outlined the challenges as well as the rewards you may experience. The following section offers a set of guided exercises designed to help the primary care partner make the rewards outweigh the worries.

First, let's take an inventory of your current situation. Go to worksheet 23 and list your five biggest worries regarding your role as primary care partner. Be honest about your areas of concern. Put down whatever comes to your mind. There are no right or wrong answers. Your worries may include many different topics: "How can I get the help I need?" "How can we manage financially?" "What if the MS progresses very quickly?"

After you've completed writing down your five biggest worries, then turn to the rewards section of the worksheet. List five things that you consider the most rewarding aspects of your role as a primary care partner. As with the worries you just listed, there are no right or wrong answers here. Rewards can vary from person to person and include things like feeling a sense of accomplishment, feeling closer to your partner, or having the opportunity to learn new skills.

WORKSHEET 23:   TAKING AN INVENTORY
OF YOUR WORRIES AND REWARDS

List your five biggest worries regarding your role as primary care partner:

1. _____

2. _____

3. _____

4. _____

5. _____

List five things that you find most rewarding in your role as primary care partner:

1. _____

2. _____

3. _____

4. _____

5. _____

After you have listed your worries and rewards, ask yourself this question: "Do the rewards outweigh the worries?" If your answer is "My rewards do not outweigh my worries," then you may find the following exercises helpful. These exercises are designed to help you reduce the strain you experience in your caring role. They are based on research that suggests that caregiver strain can be reduced by at least three factors: preparedness, easing task difficulty, and seeing eye-to-eye with your partner (Archbold and Stewart 1990).

Preparedness

We will start with preparedness. Being prepared means getting ready beforehand. It may involve becoming educated (for example, knowing what drugs are recommended for the management of MS) or developing a plan (for example, working out the details of what you and your family will do in an emergency). Go to worksheet 24 and ask yourself the questions about how well you are prepared for a number of issues related to MS.

As you answer the questions in worksheet 24, other issues may come to mind where you may think that more information or a better plan would be helpful. Jot down those issues as well. When you review your answers, pay particular attention to the items where you need more preparation. For those items, jot down potential sources of information or help you could use to develop a plan. The goal of this exercise is to help you feel more prepared to deal with day-to-day challenges of MS.

WORKSHEET 24: PREPAREDNESS FOR THE PRIMARY CARE PARTNER			
How prepared are you to	**Well-prepared**	**Need more preparation**	**Potential ways to be more prepared**
Understand what MS is?			
Understand how MS is treated by your healthcare providers?			
Understand how drugs may affect the course of MS?			
Understand how rehabilitation can help your family member function better?			
Take care of your family member's physical needs?			
Take care of your family member's emotional needs?			
Get the help you need?			
Have a handle on emergencies?			
Manage the finances?			
Arrange for health care?			
Identify resources and supports you have?			
Keep yourself emotionally/physically healthy?			
Other issues:			

Easing Task Difficulty

The next exercise involves identifying ways to make your tasks easier. Worksheet 25 contains a long list of tasks you might be doing for your partner. The list comes from research on those who provide care to family members with disabilities (Archbold and Stewart 1990; Archbold, Stewart, and Hornbrook 2001). You may not be doing all of these things, but on the other hand, there may be things you are doing that are not listed. Be sure to add them to the list.

First, check all of the activities that you assist with and then add any others that are not already on the list. Next, put a checkmark in the column labeled "Difficult" if you feel that the activity is not easy for whatever reason. Finally, for those difficult items, think about how they could be made easier. Sometimes this would involve more education. For example, if helping to transfer your family member from a bed to a chair is difficult, then having a physical therapist teach you proper techniques may make this activity easier.

In another example, many of the tasks might be easier if you had the help of a volunteer or paid caregiver to assist with driving, bathing, dressing, and so forth. Once you have completed the worksheet, you may see a pattern. Where, for example, would your life would be easier if you had help with household chores or if you had expert advice about finances or access to needed services? Getting help with a few difficult tasks may remove a considerable burden from your shoulders. Think "outside of the box" and of all the resources that may be helpful here (e.g., church groups, United Way volunteers, community volunteer Web sites, and so on).

WORSHEET 25:   MAKING YOUR TASKS EASIER

Activity	Do you help?	Difficult?	What is needed to make it easier?
Help him/her getting outside the house			
Assist with medications			
Help with eating			
Lift or transfer him/her from place to place, e.g., bed to chair			
Assist with bathing			
Assist with dressing			
Drive the car for your care partner			
Take part in leisure activities with him/her			
Help with bowel/bladder care			
Write for him/her			

Prepare meals			
Do the shopping			
Manage medical equipment, e.g., feeding tube			
Take care of his/her skin care			
Take care of finances			
Take care of legal matters			
Deal with his/her fatigue			
Deal with his/her emotional ups/downs			
Take him/her to doctors' appointments			
Take care of household maintenance			
Help him/her move around the house			
Assist in filling out forms, e.g., Social Security, insurance			
Handle his/her physical pain			
Assist with grooming			
Help him/her use the phone			
Help to handle medical emergencies			
Arrange for paid help in the home			
Help him/her to the bathroom during the night			
Other issues:			

Seeing Eye-to-Eye with Your Partner

For this final exercise, go to worksheet 26. At the top of the worksheet there is a place for you, the primary care partner, to list the top five results that you would like to come out of this caring partnership. Do this without consulting your partner. Then, have your partner with MS do the same thing. After each of you has individually listed your priorities, compare your lists. Are they alike? If not, how are they different? After you have compared them, work together to make a list that you both can agree upon.

WORKSHEET 26:   SEEING EYE-TO-EYE WITH YOUR PARTNER

For the **primary care partner,** what are the top five results that you would like to come out of this caring partnership?

1. _____

2. _____

3. _____

4. _____

5. _____

For the *partner with* MS, what are the top five results that you would like to come out of this caring partnership?

1. _____

2. _____

3. _____

4. _____

5. _____

After discussing your individual lists, what are the top five results that you mutually would like to come out of this caring partnership?

1. _____

2. _____

3. _____

4. _____

5. _____

Conclusion

Care partners are unique individuals who face ongoing challenges. Experienced care partners become experts in receiving and providing care for people with MS. The path for care partners may be bumpy and, at times, frustrating; but it also provides opportunities for joy and many of life's hidden rewards. We hope that some of the perspectives that you may have arrived at by working through this chapter may ease your journey.

CHAPTER 13

Living with Multiple Sclerosis: The Connection to Spirituality

Estelle R. Klasner, Ph.D. and Maureen Manley, MA

WHAT IS SPIRITUALITY?

This chapter will ask you to consider the influence of spirituality in your life and what, if anything, it has to do with multiple sclerosis (MS). Specifically, we will discuss definitions of spirituality within a healthcare context and the importance of spirituality in maintaining well-being. We will present the personal spiritual journey of someone who has MS, and we'll offer tools to bring you closer to your spiritual nature.

Spirituality is a very complex concept. It's hard to study and difficult to describe. One reason for this difficulty is that nearly everyone has had unique experiences that helped form his or her own understanding of spirituality. Also, as you move through life experiencing different events, spirituality takes on different meanings. A diagnosis of MS is a major life event that can and often does change the person's view of spirituality. For example, many people have reported that the diagnosis caused them to reexamine their life values and how they relate to the world around them.

Health researchers have tried to understand the spiritual dimensions of chronic illnesses. It has been widely accepted, but not well-understood, that spirituality plays an important, positive role in maintaining health for people with MS. Some healthcare professionals have defined spirituality as a set of religious beliefs. Although religious practices certainly can be included in a definition of spirituality, this type of description may be too narrow and doesn't address other approaches to spirituality.

A religious definition of spirituality ignores that segment of the population that may hold nonreligious spiritual beliefs. Healthcare researchers have also proposed broader views of spirituality that include religious and nonreligious practices. Spirituality can be defined as "our need and capacity for relationships to whatever or whoever gives meaning, purpose, and direction to our lives" (McCurdy 1998, p.82). The values that Elkins refers to include the belief that life is sacred, has meaning, and the realization that everyone and everything in the world is connected in some fashion. This broader definition of spirituality recognizes that no one size fits all approaches to spirituality.

THE CONNECTION BETWEEN SPIRITUALITY AND WELL-BEING

When we talk about MS and well-being, people tend to be surprised. Many people assume that once someone has a chronic illness like MS, that person can never be in a state of well-being. However, one of the common goals for people with MS is to achieve the highest standard of well-being possible within the context of MS. "Well-being," as it is used here, does not denote a state of perfect physical or cognitive functioning. Instead, it refers to living the best and healthiest life possible with MS. People with MS report that the ability to live well comes from a combination of three factors: competent medical care, support, and spiritual practice.

Spirituality has been identified as a health-promoting activity. It has been acknowledged that it can play a major role in the way people cope with the consequences of MS. Research has shown that spirituality can have a positive impact on the quality of life, health, and life satisfaction. A study was conducted that examined two groups of people with MS. One group reported strong spiritual practices, both religious and nonreligious. The other group reported that they did not believe or engage in spiritual activities. Measurements of general health, coping, and changes in health status were taken. Those in the group who reported strong spiritual connections demonstrated the fewest changes in health status and above-average life satisfaction and coping abilities (Sullivan 2005). Many other studies have also been done examining the connection between well-being and spirituality with similar results (McNulty et al. 2004). Generally, it has become clear that spirituality is another available tool to help people cope with the challenges of living with MS.

MAUREEN'S SPIRITUAL JOURNEY WITH MS

Maureen Manley, a world class cyclist, was at the top of her game in the early 1990s. She had spent many years training and was moving up the ladder in the cycling world. In 1994, she was better prepared than she had ever been. While cycling in a race that was going so well that Maureen thought she might be on her way to another victory, Maureen suddenly lost her vision and veered off the course. She had no idea what was happening to her.

Maureen was forced to withdraw from the race. After some rest, however, her eyesight returned. Maureen continued to cycle and she also sought medical advice about her sudden loss of eyesight and some other symptoms that she had begun to experience. Finally, a diagnosis was made. It was MS. Maureen knew that MS affected physical functioning and it had already interfered with her career goals. What could she do? How could a world-class athlete cope with MS?

That was eleven years ago! Since that time, Maureen obtained her master's degree in counseling and began working in Seattle, promoting wellness for people with MS. She has also returned to cycling.

Maureen had to redefine who she was to herself, others, and the world. She began a long spiritual journey and channeled her energies into developing the tools she needed to live well with MS, and still take part in the activities she loved. Her friendly, outgoing nature encouraged her to share her story and new identity with others who have MS. As part of Maureen's outreach to others with MS, during her lectures she often discusses the different phases of the journey that brought her to where she is today: living well with MS. She describes five distinct stages she experienced as she came to terms with MS. They were desire, acceptance, awareness, choice, and action. During the writing of this book, Maureen discussed these five stages with Dr. Klassner. The following text is based on those discussions.

Desire

Desire is the place of beginning. You've got to want to move forward to live beyond the problems that life has presented to you, while still being challenged by those problems. The desire to do that doesn't have to be a monumental occurrence; it can simply be a stirring in your soul that sparks an interest to try something new, something different, and expand your knowledge. Ultimately, it is a desire to move forward into your life.

Acceptance

Acceptance is not a place of resignation. It is the beginning. It is the place that life springs from. To be accepting means to make peace with what is, so that a greater peace may be known.

Awareness

It's so easy to be aware of what you don't want; to resist and refuse to engage with people or ideas that don't appeal to you. It's much harder to be aware of what you do want. But, if you are going to get what you want from life, you need to ask yourself how you can become aware of what you do want. One good way to start is to ask yourself these questions: "How aware am I about what I want in life?" "What do I do to make the things I want to happen actually happen?" "What do I love?" "What do I value?" "What gives meaning and purpose to my life?" "How and where are the things that give meaning and purpose to my life?" "Am I living a life that I desire, or is my life made up of reactions to the things I don't want?"

Choice

When you become aware of what you want in life, you can look at the choices you are making that create your life. Do your choices bring you more life, love, and fulfillment? How would different choices create more of what you want for yourself and those around you? How often do you repeat old choices that have predictable outcomes because you are so used to doing things the same old way? When you slow down and take a long, clear look at your life, you can try on new ideas and attitudes, and you can develop new thoughts about people, circumstances, and viewpoints about everything that has been difficult in the past.

Action

What are the actions that you are taking to create the life you desire? Ask yourself, "Does this action bring me more joy, peace, vitality, and fulfillment?" "Is this action not harmful to anyone?" If you answer yes to these questions, then your spirit is in action creating the life you yearn to live. You are living your life intentionally.

HOW YOU CAN TAKE YOUR OWN SPIRITUAL JOURNEY

Incorporating spirituality into your daily routines as a tool to live well with MS makes sense. It involves living your life with a sense of purpose. However, it isn't always easy to get started. The following section offers a number of ways to get started incorporating spiritual practices into your life as a powerful tool to use toward living the best life possible with MS.

Developing the Right Attitude

Spirituality has often been defined as a form of optimism. People who have positive life attitudes tend to live longer than those who hold more pessimistic views about life (Dello Buono, Urciuo, and DeLeo 1998). So, the first thing you need to ask yourself is this: "How can I feel more content with my life? How can I explain my having MS in a way that fits in with my view of the world?" At first, these questions may seem purely philosophical in nature. But they are not. They are extremely practical. However, to understand why they are practical, you need to decide what will help you maintain a positive attitude toward your life with MS. To get started, you can use the following worksheets to determine what would help you to establish and maintain a positive attitude.

Worksheet 27 asks you to list five things that you are sure would add more happiness to your life. The things you choose must be both realistic and attainable. For example, listing a life without MS is desirable but not attainable; so, listing it wouldn't help you maintain a positive attitude. When you've figured out five things that would make your life happier, then write short notes about how you might go about getting those things. For example, you may have always wanted to learn a foreign language, but never had the time. Now, perhaps you can make this a priority and develop a plan to make it happen. You can decide on the language you want to learn and then contact community centers in your area that may provide foreign language classes. The key is to start small so that you can make changes and see your progress.

WORKSHEET 27:   LOOKING ON THE BRIGHT SIDE

Things that would make me happier   How do I do it?

1. _____   _____

2. _____   _____

3. _____   _____

4. _____   _____

5. _____   _____

Setting Your Goals

Making sense of your MS is a fairly difficult task. Initially, it is perfectly reasonable to feel sad and overwhelmed. In order to live well, however, you need to come to terms with the diagnosis. This may require you to set new goals or think of new ways to achieve already established goals. You have to decide how MS is going to fit into your life. You cannot change MS, but you can change your attitude and behavior toward the disease and how you think about it. You need to consider MS as you make plans to reach your desired goals. This doesn't mean giving up; on the contrary, it means looking at your goals "head-on" and using your creativity and problem-solving skills to achieve those goals.

For example, suppose you've set a goal to take a yearly trip; now you need to plan your travels with your disability in mind. You can still achieve your goal, but it's likely that you'll have to take a different path to get there. Spouses, significant others, friends, counselors, medical professionals, and others may be of help in making realistic modifications or accommodations due to your MS.

In addition to making sure that your goals are attainable, you will also have to make sure your goals are manageable. An unmanageable goal, for example, might be to achieve a fully developed sense of "spiritual awareness" or "oneness" with the world. This is certainly a commendable goal, but it may be very hard to achieve. A more manageable goal might be to read an article or book about spirituality and follow its advice on how to make some positive changes in your life. Filling out worksheet 28 below would be a good first step in setting some realistic goals for yourself.

WORKSHEET 28:   SETTING REALISTIC GOALS

My immediate goals required because of MS   Goal modifications that may be

1. _____   _____

2. _____   _____

3. _____   _____

4. _____   _____

5. _____   _____

Control

Many people with MS have reported that the sense of loss of control that comes with the diagnosis is one of the hardest issues to bear and to live with. People think about control in two different ways. Some people have an *internal locus of control*, meaning they feel they can make change happen. Others have an *external locus of control*, meaning they believe things happen to them as a result of external forces. Those who have an internal locus of control are better able to handle change in their lives and make the necessary adjustments to cope with the changes.

It's true that you cannot control everything and MS certainly can cause feelings of uncertainty and unpredictability. However, you do have control over the choices you make and how you react to your circumstances. Now, take a few minutes and list several things that you feel you can control about your life. Save this list. Some time in the future, it may come in handy to remind you that you have the ability, skills, and intelligence to make things happen. When you finish making this list, you may be surprised and realize that you have more control over the events in your life than you previously thought you had.

WORKSHEET 29:   THINGS I CAN CONTROL IN MY LIFE

1. _____

2. _____

3. _____

4. _____

5. _____

HOW TO GET IN TOUCH WITH YOUR SENSE OF SPIRITUALITY

Once you've established some goals and made some decisions about what is really important to you, you need to start working on achieving your new goals. There are several resources and methods that can help you along your spiritual journey.

Your "Tool Box"

The following is a list of concrete suggestions to help you get started on your road to living well with MS. Some of these may be just what you are looking for and others may not be suitable for you at all. Use the ones you think will work and enjoy the ride!

Counseling

A diagnosis of MS is difficult to hear, and even harder to get used to. It will take you some time to adjust and move on. You may want to seek individual counseling to help you start accepting the changes in your life that having MS causes. Counseling is one way to become aware of all of your concerns and feelings and to address them. You may choose to meet with a counselor about a specific issue like your relationship with your spouse since you were diagnosed, or you may want to seek help about broader issues. Finding the right person is discussed in detail in chapter 3.

Some counselors are trained in specific techniques such as problem solving. This is a highly effective way to help people deal with chronic illness. It requires you to look at your illness and to change the way you see it to make it more tolerable. For example, you may experience a new MS symptom. Instead of immediately assuming that the disease is progressing, you can learn how to "reframe" your thoughts, and by doing that, you may realize that a new symptom is not equivalent to progression of disease. You can then take the logical step necessary to get the new treatment you may need.

Counseling can help you draw a road map and start on your journey. In the same vein, many people find that support groups, peer counselors, telephone or Web networks, and so forth are very helpful. Sharing your feelings with people who are going through similar experiences in a group or network is a good way to connect to others and the world around you. It can help you put your worries and concerns into a broader perspective when you realize there are people who understand what you are going through and are willing to help. You need to decide whether this tool is something you want to utilize.

Mind-Body Techniques

The following offers some suggestions that may help you to feel more in control of your life in small ways. Once you learn these techniques (from reading self-help books, through your therapist, etc.), you "own" them and you can call them into action at any time. One frequently used technique is called "progressive muscle relaxation."

If you are able, this method requires you to tense and relax different parts of your body, until you achieve a complete overall sense of relaxation. You tackle each part of your body separately—tensing and then relaxing the muscles of separate parts of your body, for example, your shoulders—until you've accomplished what you set out to do. If you are able to tense and relax only certain muscle groups, then concentrate on those and don't think about the areas to which you cannot apply this method.

Deep breathing is another way to get focused and promote relaxation. This is a simple technique that can be applied anywhere, anytime you think it will be of benefit. Deep breathing basically requires you to take deep breaths and hold them for progressively longer periods of time. Be aware of your physical limitations in this exercise (e.g., overexertion, spasticity issues), however; deep breathing can be used to feel calm and in control as can simply slowing your breathing.

Meditation is a very successful method for concentrating your attention totally within yourself. Meditation requires you to think only of the present moment and of your body, focusing on your breathing. You may want to use a special word or image to help you achieve a relaxed feeling. If this is something that appeals to you, practice it frequently to obtain a new sense of calm. Some people view prayer as a form of meditation.

One variation of meditation is called "guided imagery." This works especially well when you need to be distracted from an unpleasant situation. In a guided imagery meditation, you are asked to focus on an image that you associate with peace, relaxation, and control. This is particularly effective for people who must self-administer medication by injection. The individuals who practice this technique "transport" themselves to a peaceful place while they are giving themselves the injection. The injection then becomes less difficult.

Some people may need a form of guidance to learn relaxation techniques. Hypnosis has been very helpful in such situations. Hypnosis has been used successfully by many people with MS. It allows them to reach a deep state of relaxation while gaining control over mild anxiety and pain. Hypnosis doesn't cause you to feel out of control, rather it allows you to take control and concentrate on the things that you want to change. Of course, it's important to check with your physician before starting any program, and this is as true for hypnosis as it is for other mind-body techniques. Contact your local area psychological or counseling association to find board-certified hypnotists. For any of the approaches discussed above, the self-help section of a bookstore or library can be a great resource. The Internet also can provide useful guides for mind-body techniques that can teach you how to relax and thus to live more comfortably with MS.

Freeing Your Creative Energies

Some people find it quite difficult to express themselves with words. But there are many ways to express yourself. Different forms of art, writing, or music can be used as ways to explore your innermost thoughts and feelings and get in touch with your spirit. Find your unique form of self-expression and use it to make positive changes in your life. When you begin to express your creativity, you can often tap into the spiritual dimension in your life.

Conclusion

MS is a serious medical condition that changes the lives of the people who are diagnosed with it and those around them. Having MS may not be the life you imagined for yourself before your diagnosis, but you still retain the ability to take control and make the choices that will give your life purpose and meaning. For some of you, the necessity to deal with this disease sometimes results in deeper explorations of your inner life and spiritual nature than you would have undertaken if you did not have MS. Such explorations can give your life greater meaning and richness.

CHAPTER 14

Optimizing Your Love and Sex Life

Frederick W. Foley, Ph.D.

THE CHALLENGES PRESENTED BY MS

Although multiple sclerosis (MS) presents challenges, couples can learn to approach things in a head-on, problem-solving fashion and come out on the other side with success. In some cases, your sexual relationship can become even better due to the clarity of your communication.

Even when MS is a part of your relationship, everyone retains the capacity to give and receive pleasure, although, sometimes, creative problem solving is necessary to find satisfying avenues for intimate communication. Understanding how MS symptoms might affect your intimacy and sexuality needs is the first step toward becoming empowered to overcome any obstacles effectively. Whether you are newly diagnosed, physically disabled, young, mature, single, or in a committed relationship, MS does not diminish the universal human need to love and be loved.

THE FREQUENCY OF SEXUAL CHANGES IN MS

In the general population of the United States, the prevalence of sexual concerns or problems ranges from approximately 30 percent for men and up to 40 percent for women. So, it's important to understand that sexual concerns are quite common. Although normal sexual function changes throughout the life span, having MS can affect your sexuality experience in a variety of ways (Laumann and Rosen 1999).

Studies on the prevalence of sexual problems in MS indicate that between 40 to 80 percent of women and 50 to 90 percent of men have sexual complaints or concerns. The most frequently reported changes in men are diminished capacity to obtain or maintain an erection and difficulty having an orgasm. The most frequent changes that women report are a partial or total loss of libido (sexual desire), vaginal dryness/irritation, and sensory changes in the genitals (Zorzon et al. 1999).

Sexual changes in MS can be characterized as primary, secondary, or tertiary in nature. *Primary sexual dysfunction* stems from neurological changes that directly impair your sexual response and/or sexual feelings. Primary disturbances can include partial or total loss of libido, unpleasant or decreased sensations in the genitals, decreased vaginal lubrication or erectile capacity, and decreased frequency and/or intensity of orgasm. *Secondary sexual dysfunction* refers to MS-related physical changes that indirectly affect your sexual response. Bladder and/or bowel dysfunction, fatigue, spasticity, muscle weakness, problems with attention and concentration, hand tremors, and nongenital changes in sensation are included as the most common MS symptoms that can cause secondary sexual dysfunction. *Tertiary sexual dysfunction* results from psychosocial and cultural issues that can interfere with sexual feelings and sexual response. Depression, changes in family roles, lowered self-esteem, and internalized beliefs and expectations about what defines a "sexual man" or a "sexual woman," in the context of having a disability, all may contribute to tertiary sexual dysfunction.

THE CENTRAL NERVOUS SYSTEM AND SEXUAL RESPONSE

Sexual response is mediated by the central nervous system: the brain and spinal cord. There is no single sexual center in the central nervous system. Many different areas of the brain are involved in various aspects of sexual functioning, including sex drive, perception of sexual stimuli and pleasure, movement, sensation, cognition, and attention. Sexual messages are communicated between various sections of the brain, thoracic (upper), lumbar (middle), and sacral (lower) spinal cord, and genitals throughout the sexual response cycle. Since MS can result in randomly distributed lesions along many of these pathways, it is not surprising that changes in sexual function are reported so frequently. The good news is that there are likely to be neurological pathways that mediate aspects of sexual feelings and response that are not affected by MS lesions because of how widely distributed they are.

Primary, secondary, and tertiary sexual dysfunction in MS can impact each stage in the entire sexual response cycle.

The Excitement Phase of Sexual Response and MS

MS can interfere with the "excitement" phase of the sexual response cycle at primary, secondary, and tertiary levels. Lesions in the brain can interfere with the interpretation of sexual stimuli as arousing, while lesions of the spinal cord can interfere in the transmission of sexually arousing nerve signals to the genitals. Lesions in the sacral (lower) spinal cord can also cause primary sexual dysfunction, by inhibiting or preventing the inflow of blood to the sex organs, resulting in diminished or absent erections, the lack of clitoral swelling, and/or the absence of vaginal lubrication.

Fatigue can cause secondary "excitement" dysfunction by interrupting the usual capacity to interpret sexual stimuli (e.g., the sight or touch of one's sexual partner) as exciting, and by decreasing the frequency of sexual thoughts and fantasies.

Another secondary or indirect physical symptom is caused by using medications that may have an impact on your sexual response. For example, some tricyclic antidepressant medications may cause vaginal dryness, and the use of selective serotonin reuptake inhibitors (SSRIs) can cause loss of libido or difficulty having an orgasm.

Changes in role function can cause tertiary difficulties within the "excitement" phase in a number of ways. For example, if you have MS, it may be difficult to see yourself as a fully expressive sexual person, or if your sexual partner is also your primary caregiver, it may be difficult to switch from your caregiver–care receiver to sexual lover roles. This can result in loss of libido (desire). Libido sets the stage for your interpretation of potentially exciting sexual stimuli as exciting.

In addition, negative body image, depression, and feelings of dependency that may result from role changes can all negatively impact the excitement phase by interfering with your psychological processes that are necessary to feel sexually responsive.

The Plateau Phase of the Sexual Response Cycle and MS

In primary sexual dysfunction, MS lesions in the spinal cord may directly make it difficult to sustain penile and clitoral/vaginal engorgement during the plateau phase. In addition, sensory changes in the genitals can interrupt or diminish nerve signals that initiate and/or maintain vasocongestion at both the spinal cord and cerebral cortex (brain) levels. Secondary sexual dysfunction impacts the plateau phase as well. Spastic or *flaccid* (not firm) lower limbs can disturb the increase in lower body muscle tension that normally helps to build excitement during the plateau phase.

Bladder and bowel dysfunction are correlated with reports of sexual problems in MS. Nerve pathways that control the muscles of the bladder are very close to those that regulate the sexual response, and demyelinating lesions in the spinal cord and brain may affect bladder and sexual function together. In tertiary sexual dysfunction, the fear of losing bladder or bowel control during sexual activity with a partner can dramatically inhibit your sexual desire and enjoyment.

Difficulties with attention and concentration may also interfere with the plateau phase of sexual response. Sexual arousal can be sustained only with the continuous interpretation of sexual stimuli as sexually stimulating. Although subtle, impairments in attention can cause you to lose focus during the sexual experience, which can interfere with maintaining arousal. This can be frustrating for both you and your sexual partner; you can have trouble concentrating and this symptom may be interpreted by your partner as meaning that he or she is deficient as a lover.

Orgasm and MS

If you have MS, you may also report loss of orgasm as a symptom, even when the sexual experiences associated with the excitement and plateau phases seem relatively unaffected. More commonly reported are less frequent orgasms, which can result from direct physical (primary), indirect physical (secondary), or the psychosocial (tertiary) causes. In addition, when there are problems interrupting the excitement and plateau phases, the necessary physical and emotional prerequisites for orgasm may be absent.

OPTIMIZING YOUR SEX LIFE: ASSESSMENT OF SEXUAL PROBLEMS

Before you decide to discuss your sexual problems with your healthcare team, take the following test, which was developed specifically for people with MS:

WORKSHEET 30: MS SYMPTOMS AND SEXUALITY*

Over the last six months, the following MS symptoms have interfered with my sexual activity or satisfaction:	Never 0	Rarely 1	Sometimes 2	Frequently 3
Muscle tightness or spasms in my arms, legs, or body				
Bladder or urinary symptoms				
Bowel symptoms				
Feelings of dependency because of MS				
Pain, burning, or discomfort in my body				
Feeling that my body is less attractive				
Problems moving my body the way I want to during sexual activity				
Feeling less masculine or feminine due to MS				
Problems with concentration, memory, or thinking				
Less feeling or numbness in my genitals				
Fear of being rejected sexually because of MS				
Worries about sexually satisfying my partner				
Feeling less confident about my sexuality due to MS				
Lack of sexual interest or desire				
Less intense or pleasurable orgasms or climaxes				
Takes too long to orgasm or climax				
Inadequate vaginal wetness or lubrication (women)/difficulty getting or keeping a satisfactory erection (men)				

Scoring: Add the Columns   =

Total Score _____

If you scored 3 on any item, or your total score adds up to more than 6, then you should discuss your sexual issues with your MS healthcare provider.

* Note: Adapted from Sanders, A. S., F. W. Foley, N. G. LaRocca, and V. Zemon. 2000. The multiple sclerosis intimacy and sexuality questionnaire-19 [MSISQ=19]. *Sexuality and Disability* 18(1):3–26.

Your answers to the questions above will give you a place to start. Begin by discussing these issues with your partner and bring your answers to this quiz with you to your MS healthcare provider. The path to finding solutions begins by identifying what the main symptoms or problems are.

FINDING SOLUTIONS FOR CHANGES IN SEXUALITY

Unfortunately, healthcare providers rarely bring up the subject of sexuality, because of patients' personal discomfort, lack of professional training in this area on the healthcare provider's part, or fears of being overly intrusive. However, if you bring up the subject, most providers will be willing to discuss it.

Communicate Proactively with Your HealthCare Providers and Your Partner

It is critical to discuss the changes in your sexual feelings and ask directly about treatments that are available to enhance sexuality. Talk over with your doctor the ways in which your symptoms and the medications used to treat them may be affecting your sexual responses. If you have a sexual partner, bring your partner with you to the appointment, so you can begin the problem-solving process together. To become more comfortable with talking to your partner about these sensitive issues, you can use the checklist below. Which of the following activities are you doing?

Checklist 13: Becoming Comfortable with Your Sexuality

_____ Agree on when and where to talk about it; if there is a great deal of discomfort, have a professional counselor help you.

_____ Strive to understand and empathize with each other. This means avoiding blaming, accusing, or expressing your dissatisfactions with each other.

_____ Focus on clarity between the two of you for concerns about specific areas of sensation and loss, times of tiredness in the day, and other physical or cognitive concerns.

_____ Take time to touch and hug each other warmly during these discussions.

_____ Focus only on sharing information and developing the "next steps" in a plan to improve your intimate and sexual communication.

_____ Do not expect perfection. Above all else, do not forget to support each other throughout this process.

_____ Remember that MS symptoms may wax and wane. Solutions that work today may need to be revised tomorrow.

Optimizing Libido

If you are in an intimate relationship, begin by focusing on the "sensual" and "special person" aspects of your relationship. Sensual aspects include all forms of physically and emotionally pleasing nongenital contacts like back rubs and gentle stroking of nongenital body zones. During periods of diminished sex drive, you may forget to express appreciation for each other, which is one of the cornerstones of a long-term intimate relationship. The sensual, nonsexual aspects to your physical relationship can become diminished during such periods of diminished sex drive, but they are essential to maintaining emotional intimacy. To counter that possibility, make dates for nonsexual but sensual evenings. You can enjoy each other emotionally and physically and engage in enjoyable sensual exploration of each others' bodies, without the pressure of working toward sexual intercourse. Tender-hearted, simple cuddling can be delightful and very satisfying. Restore the "special person" aspects to your relationship, which include all those behaviors that demonstrate to your partner that he or she is important and very special to you. Loving gestures tend to get lost in the midst of the pressures of coping with MS symptoms and other life-survival tasks. Increasing these special acts of caring toward one another sets the stage for increasing intimacy which, in turn, sometimes stimulates new libidinous energies.

Whether you currently have a sexual partner or not, exploring your sensual and erotic body zones can be an important step in restoring diminished libido. Combining enjoyable cerebral sexual stimulation (achieved via fantasy, sexually explicit videos, books, and so forth) with masturbation or sensual physical self-exploration is sometimes helpful. Using vibrators or other sexual toys may complement these efforts.

Developing a "sensory body map" with your partner to explore the exact locations of pleasant, decreased, or altered sensations can improve intimate communication and set the stage for increasing pleasure for the two of you.

Sensory Body Mapping Exercise

- Conduct this exercise without your clothes on, in a place that is private, relaxing, and kept at a comfortable temperature.

- Begin by systematically touching your body from head to toe (or all those places you can reach comfortably).

- Vary the rate, rhythm, and pressure of your touch, allowing approximately fifteen to twenty minutes for the entire exercise.

- Note areas of sensual pleasure, discomfort, or sensory change. Alter your pattern of touch to maximize the pleasure you feel (without trying to obtain sexual satisfaction or orgasm).

- Next, inform your partner of your "body map" information and instruct him/her in touching you in a similar fashion.

- Have your partner provide the same information for you (about her/his body map). Take turns giving pleasure to each other, without engaging in sexual intercourse or trying to orgasm. Remember, the emphasis here is on communication and pleasure, not on sex or orgasm. This exercise can set the stage for you to rediscover pleasure in spite of the diminished desire caused by MS.

For women, pelvic floor (or Kegel) exercises sometimes can enhance female sexual responsiveness, although it is not known whether or not they are helpful in MS. To perform the Kegel exercises, alternately tighten and release the pubococcygeus muscle (identifiable as the muscle that starts and stops the flow of urine mid-stream). Exercising this muscle twenty-five or more times a day is recommended.

Note: Initially, it is essential to learn exactly where these muscles are located during urination. But once you know where the muscles are, it is very important to then conduct the exercise when you are *not* urinating. This is important due to the high frequency of urine retention in MS, which can lead to bladder infections.

Optimizing Sexual Pleasure with Decreased or Changed Genital Sensations

To enhance sexual response when decreased or changed genital sensations have occurred, increase stimulation to other erogenous zones, such as breasts, buttocks, ears, and lips. Conduct a sensory "body map" exercise by yourself or with your partner to explore the exact locations of pleasant, decreased, or altered sensations. Increase cerebral stimulation by watching sexually oriented videos, exploring fantasies, and introducing new kinds of sexual play into your sexual activities. As with the treatment of all sexual symptoms in MS, sexual experimentation and communication are the keys to maximizing sexual response and sexual pleasure.

Increase genital stimulation through vigorous oral stimulation or with the aid of mechanical vibrators (available by mail order). Strap-on clitoral vibrators do not interfere with intercourse and require little manipulation once in place. Vibrators that attach to the base of the penis can help to stimulate erections in men, and provide direct clitoral stimulation during intercourse.

Note that painful or irritating genital or body sensations sometimes can be treated with medications. Amitriptyline (Elavil®), carbamazepine (Tegretol®), and phenytoin (Dilantin®) are occasionally prescribed to help manage this difficult symptom.

Optimizing Erectile Function

There are a wide variety of approaches that improve erectile capacity, allowing almost all men to optimize the quality of their erections. Approaches include the following: oral medicines, injectable medicines, intraurethral and topical medicines, mechanical erectile aids, surgery, and counseling.

Medicines. Oral medicines include PDE-5 (phosphodiesterase-type-5) inhibitors. PDE-5 inhibitors work by blocking a chemical in erectile tissue that causes erections to become flaccid. These medicines include sildenafil (Viagra®), vardenafil (Levitra®), and tadalafil (Cialis®). To date, only sildenafil has been completed in its clinical trials with men who have MS, although the other medicines are highly similar and can be prescribed for people with MS. These medicines are helpful in maintaining erections, but they are not useful when the individual cannot initiate an erectile response. Typically, they are taken an hour before anticipated sexual activity. The effects of vardenafil and tadalafil are reported to last somewhat longer than sildenafil, although they have not yet been tested in men who have MS. **Caution:** These medicines cannot be used with some nitrate-based cardiac medicines, since they interact with each other and can lower blood pressure excessively.

In addition to the PDE-5 inhibitors, there are other oral medicines currently in development for erectile dysfunction that work by enhancing or blocking chemical pathways in the brain and spinal cord related to sexual function. To date, none of these medicines have been tried for individuals with MS.

Another approach involves the injection of medications into the penis, such as alprostadil (Prostin VR®) or papaverine, which cause engorgement of the penile erectile tissues. Auto-injectors are available that work with a simple push-button mechanism. The injection usually causes only mild momentary discomfort. Side effects are minimal for most users, if instructions by the urologist or prescribing physician are carefully followed.

Alprostadil can also be administered via urethral suppository (MUSE®), in addition to the penile injection. In this approach, a small plastic applicator inserts the drug into the urethra, where it is absorbed and subsequently stimulates a satisfactory erection in most men. Approximately one-third of men who have tried the drug reported some penile discomfort with its use and in rare instances *priapism* can occur (priapism is a prolonged erection that may require medical care after three hours) (Padma et al. 1997).

Mechanical aids. These are generally noninvasive and include vibrators or vacuum pumps to enhance erections. With a vacuum tube and constriction band, a plastic tube is fitted over the flaccid penis and a suction pump or tube is operated to create a vacuum to produce an erection. A latex band is slipped from the base of the tube onto the base of the penis. The band maintains engorgement of the penis for sexual activities. **Note:** The band cannot be used for more than thirty minutes. If you can attain erections easily, but have difficulty maintaining them, the constriction band alone can be used with satisfactory results.

Mail-order aids. There are a number of sexual aids available by mail order that do not require a physician's prescription. Some men prefer strap-on latex penises, some of which are hollow and can hold a flaccid or semi-erect penis. Strap-on, battery-operated vibrators in the shape of a penis are also available.

Prostheses. A more invasive form of treatment for erectile problems is the penile prosthesis. Although there are different types of prostheses, they all require surgical insertion of rods or inflatable chambers into the penis. There are greater risks associated with surgery than with other methods, such as infection, scarring, and other difficulties with the implants. Nevertheless, approximately 80 percent of men using these types of prostheses find them satisfactory. In general, a penile prosthesis is recommended only when other efforts to manage erectile dysfunction have not been successful (Brinkman et al. 2005).

Counseling. Finally, counseling is very helpful, particularly when there is performance anxiety, depression, inhibition about communication, or other tertiary sexual problems. When coping with erectile dysfunction, it is very important to include your sex partner in the discussion, if you are in a long-term relationship. This will enhance intimacy by allowing both of you to learn and explore together. If partners feel inhibited about talking through these issues, counseling with a mental health professional who is knowledgeable about MS can be helpful.

Optimizing Pleasure When Vaginal Dryness or Tightness Occurs

Similar to the erectile response in men, the vaginal lubrication response in women is controlled by multiple pathways in the brain and spinal cord. *Psychogenic lubrication* originates in the brain, and occurs through fantasy or exposure to sexually related stimuli. Establishing a relaxing, romantic, and sexually stimulating setting for sexual activity, incorporating relaxing massage into foreplay activities, and prolonging such foreplay activities can enhance psychogenic lubrication.

Reflexogenic lubrication occurs through direct stimulation of the genitals via a reflex response in the sacral (lower) part of the spinal cord. Reflexogenic lubrication sometimes can be increased by manually or orally stimulating the genitals. The simplest method to cope with vaginal dryness is to apply generous amounts of water-soluble lubricants (e.g., K-Y® jelly). Make sure you use plenty of lubricant . . . most people do not use sufficient amounts. Don't be afraid to "soak the sheets." Some women report that using vegetable oils such as corn oil (typically used for cooking) feels more soothing on vaginal tissues than water-based lubricants. Healthcare professionals do *not* advise the use of petroleum-based jellies (e.g., Vaseline®) for vaginal lubrication, because they can leave residues that could cause bacterial infections to develop.

Optimizing Pleasure When Spasticity Occurs

Spasticity in the hips or legs can make finding a comfortable position for sexual intercourse very difficult. Active management of symptoms typically includes physical therapy exercises and antispasticity medications. Administering antispasticity medication before engaging in sexual activity can be helpful. Be sure, however, to discuss any medication changes with your physician.

Another approach for coping with spasticity is to explore alternative sexual positions for intercourse. Women with spasticity of their adductor muscles may find lying on their side with the partner approaching from behind more comfortable. A man who has difficulty straightening his legs may find that sitting upright in an armless chair allows his partner to mount his erect penis. However, everyone's body is different, and the key to finding alternative sexual positions is open exploration and communication between partners.

Note: It can be very helpful to try new positions while you still have your clothes on (i.e., when you are not engaging in sexual acts), so that any anxiety you or your partner feels will be reduced and you both will not feel so vulnerable.

Optimizing Sexuality with MS-Related Fatigue

Typically, fatigue is managed from physical therapy, occupational therapy, and pharmacological perspectives. Consult your MS healthcare team about potential medicines for fatigue. Having sex in the morning or at times during the day when your energy levels are higher can compensate for fatigue. If you're tired, be honest, and you can make a date after you take a nap or for a different time of day. In addition, exploring sexual positions that minimize weight-bearing or tiring movements can minimize fatigue. Open communication and the willingness to engage in trial-and-error exploration are essential ingredients.

Optimizing Sexuality with Bladder Dysfunction

Tailoring symptomatic bladder management strategies around anticipated sexual activity is the basic approach. Proactive discussion with your sex partner and MS healthcare team minimizes the risk of incontinence during sexual activity. For example, altering your schedule for taking anticholinergic medications (frequently given for bladder storage dysfunction) to thirty minutes before anticipated sexual activity may minimize bladder contractions during sex. Because vaginal dryness increases with the use of these medicines, using water-soluble lubricants is important. Restricting your fluid intake for an hour before sex and conducting intermittent catheterization just before engaging in genital sexual activity will also minimize incontinence. Men who experience small amounts of urine leakage can wear a condom during sex.

Women who have indwelling catheters can tape the catheter securely to the stomach, empty the collecting bag before sexual activity, and put additional tape around the top ring to minimize the chances of leaks. Lying in a "nestled spoons" position with the woman in front, and using rear entry intercourse, will avoid putting pressure on the catheter or the collecting bag.

Optimizing Sexual Function with Muscle Weakness

Finding new positions for satisfactory sexual activities can compensate for weakness. Reclining positions are less tiring, pillows under the hips can improve positioning and reduce muscle strain. Oral sex requires less movement than intercourse, and using hand-held or strap-on vibrators can provide sexual satisfaction while compensating for muscle weakness. If both partners conduct a "positioning" exercise before sex, that will help them to determine whether the new positions are comfortable, without introducing anxiety during sexual activity.

Optimizing Your Sex Life When Changes in Attention and Concentration Occur

Changes in attention and concentration may derail your ability to sustain sexual interest, which may create feelings of confusion, guilt, and rejection. These negative feelings can increase distractibility, or lead you to avoid sex altogether. In general, minimizing nonromantic or nonsexual stimuli and maximizing sensual and sexual stimulation during sex is the best strategy for compensating.

Use multisensory stimulation, including talking in sexy ways, sensual and erotic touching, and playing romantic music can help to minimize this problem. When the partner with MS loses focus, briefly switching from erotic to nonerotic touching can create an atmosphere of acceptance and ease the couple back into erotic sexuality.

Sometimes, body image concerns can prove distracting, since you may tend to concentrate or focus on areas of your body or your partner's (or performance) that you're not satisfied with, rather than the pleasure you are capable of giving or receiving. If you find your thoughts drifting away from the pleasure of the moment and onto body image or other concerns, it's very important to redirect your attention back to those aspects of your body you are pleased with, or back to appreciating what you can enjoy.

Optimizing Sexuality with Depression or Other Changes in Mood

Frequently, MS is associated with clinical depression, grief, demoralization, or temporary changes in self-esteem and body image. These emotional challenges can temporarily dampen sexual interest and pleasure, especially clinical depression. Usually, medications and psychotherapy can offer relief from clinical depression, which restores sexual interest. However, a group of antidepressants called selective serotonin reuptake inhibitors (SSRIs), which include Prozac®, Paxil®, Zoloft®, and Lexipro®, can cause loss of libido or interfere with orgasm. **Note:** Before you begin any antidepressant therapy, consult your doctor about any potential sexual side effects.

Coping with Role Changes and Loss of Intimacy

Western cultural expectations about sex include the notion that sex should be spontaneous and passionate. If enculturated visions of what sex "should be" are not met, lovers may feel so disappointed that they withdraw from the sexual relationship and fail to explore or enjoy other sexual possibilities.

In Western societies, women are particularly susceptible to having a negative body image, which MS-related disabilities may exacerbate. Similarly, men with MS may view themselves as failing to live up to some internalized role such as "breadwinner," being physically strong and brave, or being the sexual initiator. Sometimes, the struggle with internalized role expectations for yourself and your partner can result in a gradual loss of seeing each other as sexually appealing.

This process can become accelerated if the "well" partner provides extensive care and assistance to the "sick" or "disabled" partner. When caregiving becomes an extensive part of a relationship, it can be difficult to relax and have sexual fun. See chapter 12 on the care partner relationship for the importance of respite for the caregiver and the importance of using many other resources for caregiving needs. A diminishing capacity to understand and work through these issues also can create greater isolation and misunderstanding, and resentments toward each other may grow (see chapter 10 for further clarification of cognitive concerns).

Obtaining educational and resource materials can facilitate helpful discussions. They are available through the National Multiple Sclerosis Society or from other resources listed at the back of this book. In addition, there are many self-help books available at most local bookstores that are designed to enhance sexual and intimate communication. Read them with your partner. Set aside time each week to talk about what you are reading, and decide whether what you've read applies to your relationship or not.

Another approach involves setting aside time each week or making actual dates, on a regular basis, to devote the time exclusively to restoring intimacy and talking about your sexuality. This can set the stage for a couple to slowly develop greater ease in talking about their sensual, sexual, and intimate desires and differences. The MS situation requires that couples "rediscover" each other, because their roles and expectations need to be updated or reconciled with the presence of MS.

Conclusion

This chapter is not meant to be exhaustive in relation to examining concerns that can affect your sexuality with MS. It is also not exhaustive in relation to strategies for improving your love and sex life, e.g., the impact of any of your medications could be important. Nevertheless, it is hoped that this chapter will provide you with a good framework for overcoming the challenges that MS may have brought into your sexual life.

CHAPTER 15

Tapping Available Community Resources

David C. Clemmons, Ph.D., C.R.C. and Nancy J. Holland, Ed.D., RN

FINDING YOUR WAY

Living with multiple sclerosis (MS) can be a demanding, sometimes overwhelming task if you try to do everything by yourself. Fortunately, there are many community resources available to you. The trick is to learn what services there are, where they are, and how best to use them. Until they are needed, you may not realize how many no-cost/low-cost resources there are in your community.

In this chapter, we discuss four subjects. First, we talk about how to find useful information. This is probably the most important part of our discussion. We try to help you figure out how to find out about services (or anything else) you want. Second, we have a short discussion about the Internet. This is really a continuation of our discussion on finding information. We try to demystify the Internet and we talk about how to use it efficiently. After all, if computers were not really "user-friendly," most people wouldn't be using them. Third, we provide a list of ideas about exploring possible resources in your community. This is meant to be a "brainstorming" list, not an exhaustive directory or even complete list. Fourth and last, we provide you with some tips and ideas for evaluating the information and agencies you find. This is sort of a "quality control" section. It reminds you, the reader, that it is important to be a wise consumer!

GETTING INFORMATION

Let's start with how to get information. You may not get the services you need simply because you haven't figured out how to get the right information about them. Furthermore, getting the right information is sometimes difficult. For instance, try looking up "garbage collection" in your telephone book. In many phone books, it is listed under "solid waste disposal." How would you know this if you were from a different country or even a different city? If you don't know the right terms to use (or someone who does), your garbage might never get picked up. Most information about nearly every aspect of our culture is listed somewhere. The trick is finding out where it is and the easiest way to get it.

Libraries

Thanks to Benjamin Franklin (and Andrew Carnegie), public libraries are one of the most useful and most user-friendly sources for information. Libraries are not just collections of books, videos, and CDs. They are good resources for finding out about community services, if you know how to go about it. Fortunately, you don't have to be a library expert to use a library. Librarians and library staff are in excellent locations for finding out about community resources, and they enjoy working on information requests and helping people to use library tools. The sister of one of the authors of this chapter is a librarian. She convinced us to start our discussion about community services by talking about libraries first, because libraries provide the most consistently valuable resource for information for everyone in our country.

Some large libraries, such as those in Seattle, Boston, and Baltimore, actually have whole departments exclusively devoted to providing people with information over the telephone. The program in Seattle is called "Quick Information" and is nationally known for its excellence. People call these libraries to ask any informational question that is important enough to them to want an answer. A large portion of these calls are requests for how to find help through service agencies or other local sources, e.g., "I need to find a support group for people with Parkinson's condition" or "Can you help me find information about employment discrimination?" Even if a library close to you doesn't have a department devoted specifically to providing callers with information, it's more than likely the librarians will be good at helping you find what you need. Sometimes, all you have to do is know how to ask for what you need.

It's been our experience that almost all of the librarians and support staffs with whom we work enjoy helping others to explore new areas of information. It's also a good idea to let library staff know how much you appreciate their help. Those of us who work with library personnel see them as part of our support network and we let them know how much their help is valued. After all, what better people can you think of to help you find information than the professionals who specialize in disseminating information?

County and Municipal Information Sources

In many instances, especially in more rural areas, you'll have to think out of the box a bit to find formal and informal networks that might have answers to your needs. Your local Chamber of Commerce can be an excellent resource, as can many local religious facilities. Most cities and towns have a social service office that can explain your needs to other municipal departments that, in turn, can help you if you have special concerns. Many agencies and government departments have specialized services for senior citizens (people over the age of fifty-five), veterans, or people with physical disabilities or other limitations.

Don't neglect fraternal organizations or service organizations, like the Rotary, Lions, or Kiwanis clubs. Ask a member to take you to a meeting and make your need known. Some of these fraternal groups run small grant programs for health, vision, or dental care and other types of aid. Don't forget to check out your area newspapers, free throwaway weeklies, or end-of-the-week supplements with calendars that list events and activities. You can find anything in these from classes on job-seeking to free services, to announcements of upcoming plays, and so on. Finally, don't forget informal forums, such as the local barbershop, gas station, hair salon, coffee shop, and so forth. These meeting places provide very valuable and, at times, the only local human networks.

Of course, getting information doesn't help you very much unless you are able to store it in a format where you can get to it quickly when you need it. So, here is a short checklist that you can use to quiz yourself about important strategies for storing and keeping information:

Checklist 14: Saving Information Records

____ Do I have a plan for recording all of my agency contacts by date? (See the Format for Record Keeping below.)

____ Do I have permanent storage for all records I make?

____ Do I keep duplicate records of important information?

____ If I am using a computer, do I back up my information (that is, on a floppy disk or tape)?

____ If I am disorganized and can't keep track of my papers and affairs, do I have a close friend or family member who is willing to check or keep duplicate backup records for me?

Do you already have a format for storing or organizing important information? The following checklist provides the points to consider when you are organizing information and offers a useful structure for storing it.

Checklist 15: Format for Record Keeping

1. **Important instruction:** When you decide on a record keeping format, make sure you always keep and file your records in the same way, each time you add something to a file. For records of your dealings with social service agencies, the following items should always be recorded and kept on file:

2. Date of agency contact

3. Name of agency

4. Mailing address/physical address (not always the same)

5. Electronic addresses: e-mail address; Web site; fax number; and telephone number

6. Name of specific contact person (first and last names)

7. Brief comment about results

8. What to do next? (very important)

USING THE INTERNET

Now, let's move on to the Internet, also called the "Web" or the "Net." Looking for information on the Internet is sometimes called "surfing the Net." We don't have the space to teach you how to surf the Net. We can, however, offer some suggestions about using a computer to find community resources.

First, if you don't know how to use a computer, the good news is that it is fairly easy to learn how to operate one. Second, if you don't have a computer, many libraries offer free computer access to people who have library cards. It wouldn't be fair to ask library staff to teach you how to use the computer, but when we researched this article, it became clear that the library is an excellent place to find out where inexpensive or free computer classes can be located in your area. In rural areas (or even in some urban areas), if the librarian has the time, you may get some free lessons. Using a computer is just like learning to drive: once you learn the basics, the rest is just practice.

How to Do a Computer Search

Suppose you want to do a computer search about a subject that interests you. First, of course, you have to know the basics, like how to turn on the computer, and how to find a search engine to conduct your search. If you are using a public computer as at a library, you probably won't even have to turn it on. Often, the librarian or a staff member will guide you in this procedure. Once the computer has been turned on, you need only do the following:

1. Open a search engine, which is a free service that helps you look for information. Currently, the name of the most well-known search engine is "Google." If you are using a library computer, it's more than likely the computer will have Google available for your use. It's very easy to learn how to use. Remember, if the computer were not user-friendly, it would not be used by so many people.

2. Enter some "key words" into the search engine. Key words are words that are likely to be included in information you are seeking. For example, if you're looking for alternative medical approaches to multiple sclerosis, you would type in the words "alternative medicine" and the words "multiple sclerosis."

3. Usually, it's best to insert quotation marks (" ") around the words that belong together. This way, the computer will search for and find only the combination of the words you want. In the example above, you want to find every instance of the term "alternative medicine." You don't want to find every instance of the word "alternative" and every instance of the word "medicine."

4. After you enter your key words, hit the Enter key and your search has begun.

While we were writing this chapter, we followed the steps outlined above. The computer found 331,756 different articles when we used "multiple sclerosis" and "alternative medicine." We didn't look at each article, but the first twenty-five or thirty were very interesting.

Just for fun, we also entered the words without using quotation marks. We got back more than half a million different articles. Some of them were interesting, but some didn't have anything to do with multiple sclerosis or alternative medicine. That was because the computer looked for every article that contained the separate words "medicine," "multiple," "alternative," and "sclerosis" instead of just the combinations "multiple sclerosis" and "alternative medicine." We hope that knowing these facts about the ease of doing computer searches will encourage you to do some searches on your own to find the resources and services you may need in your own community.

SPRINGBOARD RESOURCE LIST

Now, let's look at some resources that should be available to you in your community. This following is a list of agencies you might find helpful to contact for aid in dealing with any of the many issues that MS may have brought into your life.

The National Multiple Sclerosis Society (NMSS). This is probably the best MS-specific contact in the United States. See the Resources section at the back of the book for their Web address. This organization can provide general and specific information about MS. For example, they can supply you with information about employment, life planning and independence, facts for the newly diagnosed, educational and training programs, local support and educational groups, and MS-related literature. Through their local chapters NMSS offers referrals to neurologists who specialize in MS and other healthcare services, social services, legal services, and they can help you to access local government agencies, such as state rehabilitation and state employment offices. You can use NMSS as a resource for questions concerning medication, assistive devices, counseling agencies, and so forth. They can help you find practitioners of physical, occupational, speech, recreational therapies, and similar resources.

Other Web sites of interest to those with MS are also listed in the Resources section at the back of the book.

Local not-for-profit MS agencies. In addition to local chapters of NMSS, many areas also have other MS agencies that provide a variety of services. These may be statewide agencies, or agencies that focus on a smaller local area, such as a county or a region.

Legal aid/attorneys' associations. These organizations sometimes provide no-cost ("pro bono") or low-cost legal services for people who need legal help but cannot afford it. Unfortunately, these organizations are more readily available in urban areas than in rural or semirural places. But don't be afraid to call a local lawyer to ask about free consultations (pro bono work), sliding-scale fees, or a payment plan for legal services if you really need them.

Credit and debt counseling agencies. As someone with MS who may have been caught in mid-career with high credit-card debt and expensive mortgage payments, who would benefit from negotiated lower rates, consolidated debt payments, extended payment schedules, and so forth, these agencies can be invaluable to you. There are even nonprofit agencies of this type that may have no fees or low fees. **Note:** It is very important to understand the fee structure if there is one.

Federal and State Agencies

The intent of this section is to give you brief profiles of some state and federal agencies that can assist you as they have others with MS. Again, your local librarian or a search on the Internet can help you find even more options of this type.

Equal Employment Opportunity Commission (EEOC). Workers who believe that no effort was made by their employer to provide suitable accommodations for them on the job so that they would have been able to continue working in spite of having MS, or perceive that they were otherwise discriminated against should contact the EEOC. The agency representative will decide if your case has a legal basis before the EEOC engages in actual litigation. Many private lawyers won't take a discrimination case unless a finding of discrimination is made by the EEOC. This can be a time-consuming and lengthy process if you use only federal lawyers; on the other hand, if you have the resources or a new job, why not pursue it? In some cases, employment discrimination cases can be handled more expediently by a state human rights commission (or an agency with a similar title).

U.S. Department of Justice or Office of Civil/Human Rights. Clients can be referred directly to this agency for diverse types of human rights violations and discrimination issues. Depending on the volume of cases, and other matters, local county or city human rights agencies may be better at expediting a case more quickly.

AmeriCorps. This agency offers a stipend to its participants, who generally work in schools or not-for-profit agencies involved in a variety of social service enterprises. This program is very similar to the earlier federal VISTA program. The stipend is approximately $850 per month, but it can vary.

Participation in the AmeriCorps program does not count as substantial gainful activity (SGA) with respect to Social Security Disability Income (SSDI) payments. So if you receive some SSDI income, AmeriCorps can provide some useful supplementary income. The accompanying educational benefits, which can reach up to $4,725 annually (in early 2005), can be applied to further your education. Examples of AmeriCorps positions might include a high-school volunteer coordinator, a nonprofit agency marketing position, an elementary school literacy counselor, and so forth.

Vocational rehabilitation. The goal of state vocational rehabilitation agencies is to help those with disability barriers to employment become employed or reemployed. They can provide access to a variety of educational, training, and counseling services, as well as assistive technology and other services related to becoming employed. In the United States, each of the fifty states has a state rehabilitation agency. See chapter 7 for a fuller discussion of this agency.

State health and human services agencies. As with vocational rehabilitation, these agency offices are usually accessible with local offices. They provide varying amounts of basic financial subsidies, food stamps, and medical coverage if the client has no other means of support and during the long wait for Social Security eligibility to be determined.

Housing authorities. These agencies vary as to their availability on a county or city level, but they may have low-income housing available provided by the city or under Federal Section 8 availability. Rent for Section 8 housing is assessed on a graduated scale, which is determined according to the person's income. If housing will be needed in the future (i.e., if you are anticipating the loss of your home or difficulty with your rent payments), application should be made as soon as possible as a long wait period is often experienced for desirable low-cost housing.

Aging and disability services. Although the title may vary, this type of state agency usually provides different critical support services, such as "meals on wheels" deliveries, in-home care, daytime recreation programs for seniors and for those of you with significant disabilities. If you have a limited income, this type of agency can be critical both in keeping you healthy and in helping you to live independently.

Additional Service Resources

Transportation. These types of services are usually more available on a city or county level. Transportation can be a very critical service if you can no longer drive or afford the upkeep of a car, and so forth. Transportation services range from a deeply discounted bus pass to specialty van or small bus pickup services. Some communities issue taxi script that can be used in place of cash to pay for transportation by taxi.

Faith-based agencies. Islamic, Jewish, Catholic, other Christian, Mormon, and various other religious communities frequently have well-developed social service programs, funded by their respective congregations. The Church of Latter Day Saints, for instance, offers a variety of social services, often including vocational services, through the local bishop. Our experience has been that many of these religious groups have been generous in providing services for nonmembers as well as members. Services have even included emergency rent and short-term help with utility payments (e.g., the Salvation Army and St. Vincent de Paul). Don't forget this option. It can be extremely helpful.

Previously, we discussed organizing and storing information. In the following checklist, we offer some suggestions about how to approach the agencies we've described throughout this chapter to maximize your experience.

Checklist 16: Contacting Agencies

_____ Have I called and made a specific appointment for services?

_____ Will I arrive on time or early?

_____ Am I prepared? Do I have accurate, appropriate background information about my medical condition, financial needs, job résumé, and so on, relating to the purpose of my visit?

_____ Will I record exactly with whom I spoke and contact information for that person?

_____ Do I know the next steps for myself and for the agency person? Timelines?

_____ Do I understand the costs for these services, if any?

_____ If I am being teamed up with a special program (e.g., advocacy, vocational, etc.), have I checked out their references and outcomes? Can I talk to others who received this service?

QUALITY CONTROL: BEING AN INFORMED CONSUMER

Let's say you are getting quite skilled at finding potential services. You must also remember the saying, "Don't believe everything you read (see, hear, find on the Internet)." A famous saying during the Revolutionary War was: "Trust in God, but keep your powder dry." This suggests the importance of your responsibility to look out for yourself. Quality control is an important responsibility you need to accept. Not every information source has the best information, or even your best interests at heart.

You need to be more than a consumer. You need to be an informed consumer. An informed consumer is one who is good at evaluating the resources that she or he finds. This way you are more likely to avoid making poor decisions about services or having anyone take advantage of your lack of experience in choosing services. Most people would probably agree that federal, state, and other governmental agencies are usually providing services in good faith (even if they make political jokes). This may not always be the case with, for example, private-for-profit agencies or even some nonprofit agencies.

Specialists who provide rehabilitation services have had the experience of working with clients with MS who enrolled in expensive vocational programs that did not provide the expected result (a job, or marketable skills). It has even happened that services were knowingly provided that were not likely to benefit the client. It doesn't really matter what went wrong if you are stuck with a large debt for services that did not improve your life.

The more of your money and time involved, the more important it is to take your time when making decisions, whether your decision is in regard to a consumer debt agency or a training program. This statement also holds true for organizations that allow you to pay "part now, part later" or that help you get private or government loans to cover their high fees. Some "advocacy" agencies that you may think provide a free service actually can involve legal fees—to be paid by you. Even programs or agencies that do not present themselves as a fee-for-service business may have hidden costs.

The following checklist will give you some ideas about how to screen different agencies to see whether they are the best agency for you to approach.

Checklist 17: Contacting Agencies—Additional Information

1. Is this a government agency or a nongovernmental agency? _____

2. Is it a nonprofit or a for-profit agency? _____

3. Have I asked about fees and costs? This is important no matter what kind of agency (profit, nonprofit, government, nongovernment, etc.). _____

4. If the agency asks me to sign a contract, can I take it home to read carefully and discuss with friends or family? _____

5. If I sign a contract for services (i.e., like training classes), do I have to pay the full fee if I drop out early? What allowances are made? _____

6. If I am working with a "for-profit" agency or individual, have I been a good consumer by comparing options and reviewing my choices with a close friend or relative? _____

Conclusion

In this final chapter, we've talked about services in the community that may be available to those of you with MS. We discussed how to find information about these services. The Internet was specifically discussed because this is a very efficient way for people to find information. The Resources section at the end of the book provides many useful Web sites. We also talked about how to store information and how to organize it. Finally, we reviewed strategies for evaluating different agencies and making sure that the agency or individuals that you approach will provide you with the services you want. Researching and storing information about the services that may be available to you (on a computer, in a notebook, etc.) is one excellent way to plan ahead and give you more control over the life problems that sometimes occur with MS.

APPENDIX A

Work Experience Survey

Note: Appreciation is extended to Dr. Richard Roessler and the Arkansas Rehabilitation Research and Training Center staff for the use of this survey instrument. All users of the instrument need to maintain the page referencing by Dr. Roessler and the Arkansas Rehabilitation Research and Training Center. Essential accommodation sections of the survey, that is, sections II–IV and VI, are presented here.

WORK EXPERIENCE SURVEY (WES)

Section II: Accessibility: Check (✓) any problems you have getting to, from, or around on your job. List any other accessibility problems not included in the list. Describe solutions for your two most important accessibility barriers.

_____ Parking	_____ Bathrooms	_____ Temperature
_____ Public walks	_____ Water fountains	_____ Ventilation
_____ Passenger loading zones	_____ Public telephone	_____ Hazards
_____ Entrance	_____ Elevators	_____ Identification signs/labels
_____ Stairs/Steps	_____ Lighting	_____ Access to personnel offices
_____ Floors/Floor covering	_____ Warning devices	_____ Access to general use areas
_____ Seating/Tables	_____ Evacuation routes	

List any other accessibility problems:

#1 _____

#2 _____

Describe solutions for your two most important accessibility barriers:

#1 _____

#2 _____

Section III: Essential job functions: Check (✓) any essential job functions or conditions* that pose problems for you. Describe the two most important job modifications that you need, e.g., modifying existing equipment, adding new technology, or changing the type of work you do.

Physical Abilities

_____ Working 8 hours

_____ Standing all day

_____ Standing part of the time

_____ Some kneeling

_____ Some stooping

_____ Some climbing

_____ Much pulling

_____ Much pushing

_____ Much talking

_____ Seeing well

_____ Hearing well

_____ Handling

_____ Using left leg

_____ Using both hands

_____ Using both legs

_____ Using left hand

_____ Using right hand

_____ Using right leg

_____ Lifting over 100 lbs.

Lifting 51–100 lbs.

Cognitive Abilities

_____ Immediate memory

_____ Short-term memory

_____ Long-term memory

_____ Judgment: Interpersonal

_____ Thought processing

_____ Remembering

_____ Problem solving

_____ Planning

_____ Organizing

Task-Related Abilities

_____ Repetitive work

_____ Work pace/sequencing

_____ Variety of duties

_____ Read written instructions

_____ Able and licensed to drive

_____ Perform under stress/deadlines

_____ Little feedback on performance

_____ Attain precise standards/limits

_____ Follow specific instructions

_____ Writing

Social Abilities

_____ Working alone

_____ Working around others

_____ Working with others

_____ Supervising others

_____ Working with hostile others

Working Conditions

_____ Too hot

_____ Too cold

_____ Temperature changes

_____ Too wet

_____ Too humid

_____ Slippery surface

_____ Obstacles in path

_____ Dust

_____ Fumes

_____ Odors

_____ Noise

_____ Outdoors

_____ Sometimes outdoors

_____ Always inside

____ Lifting 26–50 lbs.	____ Remembering	**Company Policies**
____ Lifting 11–25 lbs.	____ Speaking/communicating	____ Inflexible work schedule
____ Lifting 0–10 lbs.	____ Initiating work activities	____ No accrual of sick leave
Raising arms above shoulders	____ Use telephone	____ Lack of flextime
____ Prolonged sitting		____ No "comp" time
		____ Inflexible job description
		____ Vague job description
		____ Infrequent reviews of job descriptions
		____ Rigid sick/vacation leave policies

Describe the two job modifications that would be most helpful to you, e.g., restructuring of the job, modification of work schedules, reassignment to another position, modification of equipment, or provision of reader and interpreters:

#1 _____

#2 _____

Section IV: Job mastery: Check (✓) any concerns* that affect your success in completing the following tasks. Describe one solution for each of your two most important concerns.

1. Getting the job done.

    ____ Believing that others think I do a good job.

    ____ Understanding how my job fits into the "big picture," i.e., the meaning of my job.

    ____ Knowing what I need to know to do my job.

    ____ Having what I need to do my job (knowledge, tools, supplies, equipment).

2. Fitting into the workforce.

    ____ Scheduling and planning my work ahead of time.

    ____ Working mostly because I like the job.

    ____ Doing a good job.

    ____ Willing to make changes when necessary.

---

* Selected items from the Career Mastery Inventory. Used with permission of the author, John O. Crites, Crites Career Consultants, Boulder, Colorado.

3. Learning the ropes.

_____ Knowing who to go to if I need help.

_____ Understanding company rules and regulations.

_____ Knowing my way around work.

_____ Feeling a "part" of what is going on at work.

4. Getting along with others.

_____ Eating lunch with friends at work.

_____ Having many friends at work.

_____ Looking forward to seeing my friends at work.

_____ Knowing what is expected of me socially on the job.

5. Getting ahead.

_____ Having a plan for where I want to be in my job in the future.

_____ Understanding what I have to do to get promoted.

_____ Knowing what training to complete to improve chances for promotion.

_____ Talking with supervisor about what I need to get promoted.

6. Planning the next career step.

_____ Considering what I will do in the future.

_____ Knowing what the opportunities are in this company.

_____ Wanting to become more specialized in my job.

_____ Having a good idea of how to advance in this company.

Describe one solution for each of your two most important job mastery concerns:

#1 _____

#2 _____

Section VI. Review Sections II–IV of the WES and list the three most significant barriers to success in your work. Describe their solutions and people/resources who can help. Be specific.

Barrier 1: _____

Solution? _____

_____

Who can help? How can they help? _____

_____

Barrier 2: _____

    Solution? _____

    _____

    Who can help? How can they help? _____

    _____

Barrier 3: _____

    Solution? _____

    _____

    Who can help? How can they help? _____

    _____

U.S. Department of Labor
Employment Standards

Wage and Hour Division
Washington, DC 20210

STATEMENT OF PRINCIPLE

The U.S. Department of Labor and community-based rehabilitation organizations are committed to the continued development and implementation of individual vocational rehabilitation programs that will facilitate the transition of persons with disabilities into employment within their communities. This transition must take place under conditions that will not jeopardize the protections afforded by the Fair Labor Standards Act to program participants, employees, employers, or other programs providing rehabilitation services to individuals with disabilities.

GUIDELINES

When ALL of the following criteria are met, the U.S. Department of Labor will NOT assert an employment relationship for purposes of the Fair Labor Standards Act.

- Participants will be individuals with physical and/or mental disabilities for whom competitive employment at or above the minimum wage level is not immediately obtainable and who, because of their disability, will need intensive ongoing support to perform in a work setting.

- Participation will be for vocational exploration, assessment or training in a community-based placement work site under the general supervision of rehabilitation organization personnel.

- Community-based placement will be clearly defined components of individual rehabilitation programs developed and designed for the benefit of each individual. The statement of needed transition services established for the exploration, assessment or training components will be included in the person's Individualized Written Rehabilitation Plan (IWRP).

- Information obtained in the IWRP will not have to be made available, however; documentation as to the individual's enrollment in the community-based placement program will be made available to the Department of Labor. The individual and, when appropriate, the parent or guardian of each individual, must be fully informed of the IWRP and the community-based placement component and have indicated voluntary participation with the understanding that participation in such a component does not entitle the participant to wages.

- The activities of the individuals at the community-based placement site does not result in an immediate advantage to the business. The Department of Labor will look at several factors.

  1. There has been no displacement of employees, vacant positions have not been filled, employees have not been relieved of assigned duties, and the individuals are not performing services that, although not ordinarily performed by employees, clearly are of benefit to the business.

  2. The individuals are under continued and direct supervision by either representatives of the rehabilitation facility or by employees of the business.

  3. Such placements are made according to the requirements of the individual's IWRP and not to meet the labor needs of the business.

  4. The periods of time spent by the individuals at any one site or in any clearly distinguishable job classification are specifically limited by the IWRP.

- While the existence of an employment relationship will not be determined exclusively on the basis of the number of hours, as a general rule, each component will not exceed the following limitations:

Vocational exploration	5 hours per job experienced
Vocational assessment	90 hours per job experienced
Vocational training	120 hours per job experienced

An employment relationship will exist unless *all of the criteria* described in the policy are met. If an employment relationship is found to exist, the business will be held responsible for full compliance with the applicable sections of the Fair Labor Standards Act, including those relating to child labor.

Business and rehabilitation organizations may, at any time, consider participants to be employees and may structure the program so that the participants are compensated in accordance with the requirements of the Fair Labor Standards Act. Whenever an employment relationship is established, the business may make use of the special minimum wage provisions provided pursuant to section 14(c) of the Act.

—Donald J. Hinkel, Chair
   National Rehabilitation Facilities Coalition
   U.S. Department of Labor

—Karen R. Keesling, Acting Administrator
   Wage and Hour Division

Employer Incentives for Hiring a Worker with a Disability

Nonpaid 215 Hour Job Tryout: This program waives the Department of Labor requirement for an individual to be compensated for work performed within a for-profit private industry. The program allows a person with a disability to work for five hours in exploration of a particular job, ninety hours to assess a participant's skill level in performing the job, and an additional 120 hours for the employer to offer the participant training for the lack of skill identified in the ninety hour assessment, for a total of 215 hours. Industrial insurance is paid through the Vocational Services Unit.

Work Opportunity Tax Credit (WOTC): This is a national program that offers employers of a program's client a tax credit for employing the person. This tax credit is based on 35 percent of the first $6,000 (up to $2,100) that the employer pays the participant. A two-page "fill in" form for this program must be signed and dated on the first day of employment and then submitted to a state tax credit unit. Information on this process can always be received from a state vocational rehabilitation agency.

On-the-Job Training: This program is operated in collaboration with a state's vocational rehabilitation agency. The program offers employers compensation to offset the costs of training the participant for a job. The formula for the compensation is based upon reimbursing about one-half of the participant's wage for a period of time (usually three months) during which the participant is offered training in a specific position. The formula can vary with more money being offered "up front" (e.g., 75 percent) and less at the end.

Selective Certification (Piece Rate): Participant's productivity is compared to other workers performing the same job duties. The participant's productivity is then compared against the hourly wage for 100 percent production. If a participant's productivity is 50 percent of other workers and the wage is $12 per hour, for example, the participant's wage would be established at $6 per hour (50 percent of $12 = $6). This rate can be reexamined if the participant's productivity increases.

Job Coaching/Coworker as Mentor: State vocational rehabilitation will often pay for this training or mentoring service while a person learns and adapts on a job.

Barrier Removal Tax Credits and Deductions: Under the Americans with Disabilities Act, in order to enable a small business to remove barriers for individuals with disabilities, provide interpreters, and modify or acquire helpful equipment, Section 44 of the Internal Revenue Code has been changed to allow a general business tax credit of up to $5,000 annually. Additionally, Section 190 of the Code allows a deduction of up to $15,000 annually to any business making qualified architectural or transportation barrier removals that improve business access for people with disabilities.

Important Federal Regulations Relating to Multiple Sclerosis and Claims for Disability Benefits from the Social Security Administration

When considering whether your MS meets the definition of "disability," the Social Security Administration will consider whether your medical records prove your MS is *so* severe that it is said to "meet the Listing of Impairments." The Listing of Impairments is a set of detailed regulations describing specific medical findings of many different medical conditions. Most people who are found disabled don't meet these seven more severe medical listings and are found disabled based on the more general definition of disability described in chapter 11. However, if your condition is proven to meet the "Listing" for MS, then, in theory, you should be found to be "disabled" immediately. Of course proving all of this is at the heart of the matter. Even if your MS does not "meet the Listing," it is important to know what medical evidence is of particular interest to Social Security in every MS claim.

"Listing of Impairments" Multiple Sclerosis
(20 CFR Appendix I to Subpart P of Part 404)
(Introduction to "The Listing" regarding Multiple Sclerosis)

E. Multiple Sclerosis. The major criteria for evaluating impairment caused by multiple sclerosis are discussed in Listing 11.09. Paragraph A provides criteria for evaluating disorganization of motor function and gives reference to 11.04B (11.04B then refers to 11.00C). Paragraph B provides references to other listings for evaluating visual or mental impairments caused by multiple sclerosis. Paragraph C provides criteria for evaluating the impairment of individuals who do not have muscle weakness or other significant disorganization of motor function at rest, but who do develop muscle weakness with activity as a result of fatigue.

Use of the criteria in 11.09C is dependent upon (1) documenting a diagnosis of multiple sclerosis, (2) obtaining a description of fatigue considered to be characteristic of multiple sclerosis, and (3) obtaining evidence that the system has actually become fatigued. The evaluation of the magnitude of the impairment must consider the degree of exercise and the severity of the resulting muscle weakness.

The criteria in 11.09C deal with motor abnormalities which occur on activity. If the disorganization of motor function is present at rest, paragraph A must be used, taking into account any further increase in muscle weakness resulting from activity.

Sensory abnormalities may occur, particularly involving central visual acuity. The decrease in visual acuity may occur after brief attempts at activity involving near vision, such as reading. This decrease in visual acuity may not persist when the specific activity is terminated, as with rest, but is predictably reproduced with resumption of the activity. The impairment of central visual acuity in these cases should be evaluated under the criteria in Listing 2.02, taking into account the fact that the decrease in visual acuity will wax and wane.

Clarification of the evidence regarding central nervous system dysfunction responsible for the symptoms may require supporting technical evidence of functional impairment such as evoked response tests during exercise.

11.09 Multiple sclerosis.

With:

A. Disorganization of motor function as described in 11.04B; or

B. Visual or mental impairment as described under the criteria in 2.02, 2.03, 2.04, or 12.02; or

C. Significant, reproducible fatigue of motor function with substantial muscle weakness on repetitive activity, demonstrated on physical examination, resulting from neurological dysfunction in areas of the central nervous system known to be pathologically involved by the multiple sclerosis process.

11.04 Central nervous system vascular accident. With one of the following more than 3 months post-vascular accident.

A. Sensory or motor aphasia resulting in ineffective speech or communication; or

B. Significant and persistent disorganization of motor function in two extremities, resulting in sustained disturbance of gross and dexterous movements, or gait and station (see 11.00C).

(Section 11.00C)

Persistent disorganization of motor function in the form of paresis or paralysis, tremor or other involuntary movements, ataxia and sensory disturbances (any or all of which may be due to cerebral, cerebellar, brain stem, spinal cord, or peripheral nerve dysfunction) which occur singly or in various combinations, frequently provides the sole or partial basis for decision in cases of neurological impairment. The assessment of impairment depends on the degree of interference with location and/or interference with the use of fingers, hands and arms.

(Section 11.00D)

In conditions which are episodic in character, such as multiple sclerosis or myasthenia gravis, consideration should be given to frequency and duration of exacerbations, length of remissions, and permanent residuals.

12.02 Organic mental disorders. Psychological or behavioral abnormalities associated with a dysfunction of the brain. History and physical examination or laboratory tests demonstrate the presence of a specific organic factor judged to be etiologically related to the abnormal mental state and loss of previously acquired functional abilities.

The required level of severity for these disorders is met when the requirements in both A and B are satisfied, or when the requirements in C are satisfied.

A. Demonstration of a loss of specific cognitive abilities or affective changes and the medically documented persistence of at least one of the following:

   1. Disorientation to time and place; or

   2. Memory impairment, either short-term (inability to learn new information), intermediate, or long-term (inability to remember information that was known some time in the past); or

   3. Perceptual or thinking disturbances (e.g., hallucinations, delusions); or

   4. Change in personality; or

   5. Disturbance in mood; or

   6. Emotional lability (e.g., explosive temper outbursts, sudden crying, etc.) and impairment in impulse control; or

   7. Loss of measured intellectual ability of at least 15 IQ points from premorbid levels or overall impairment index clearly within the severely impaired range on neuropsychological testing, e.g., Luria-Nebraska, Halstead-Reitan, etc.;

AND

B. Resulting in at least two of the following:

   1. Marked restriction of activities of daily living; or

   2. Marked difficulties in maintaining social functioning; or

   3. Marked difficulties in maintaining concentration, persistence, or pace; or

   4. Repeated episodes of decompensation, each of extended duration;

OR

C. Medically documented history of a chronic organic mental disorder of at least 2 years' duration that has caused more than a minimal limitation of ability to do basic work activities, with symptoms or signs currently attenuated by medication or psychosocial support, and one of the following:

1. Repeated episodes of decompensation, each of extended duration; or

2. A residual disease process that has resulted in such marginal adjustment that even a minimal increase in mental demands or change in the environment would be predicted to cause the individual to decompensate; or

3. Current history of 1 or more years' inability to function outside a highly supportive living arrangement, with an indication of continued need for such an arrangement.

2.02 Impairment of visual acuity. Remaining vision in the better eye after best correction is 20/200 or less.

2.03 Contraction of peripheral visual fields in the better eye.

A. To 10 or less from the point of fixation; or

B. So the widest diameter subtends an angle no greater than 20 degrees; or

C. To 20 percent or less visual field efficiency.

2.04 Loss of visual efficiency. The visual efficiency of the better eye after best correction is 20 percent or less. (The percent of remaining visual efficiency is equal to the product of the percent of remaining visual acuity efficiency and the percent of remaining visual field efficiency.)

General Considerations for Medical Reports in a Social Security Claim

1. A background or short description of the health care providers' qualifications.

2. Length of treatment history with patient and frequency of contact.

3. A description of the diagnosis of impairment suffered by the patient.

4. A discussion of the nature of the client's condition and the medical findings that support the diagnosis.

5. A review and analysis of any test results that further confirm the diagnosis and the nature of the patient's condition.

6. An interpretation of all the findings and test results and diagnosis in terms of the functional limitations imposed by the conditions on the patient's ability to work in a substantial gainful manner. Consider the following:

   ■ Ability to perform work activities on a sustained regular and continuing basis.

- If appropriate, the impact of health problems on patient's ability to sit, stand, walk, lift, carry, push, pull, or other physical limitations.

- If appropriate, limitations on the patient's ability to understand, carry out, and remember instructions, use judgment in making work-related decisions, respond appropriately to supervision, coworkers, and work situations, and deal with changes in a routine work setting.

- If appropriate, any postural, manipulative, visual, or communicative limitations.

7. Conditions drawn by a treating health care provider with respect to a patient's limitations and work abilities will be generally disregarded unless the conclusions are explained.

Information provided by:
Kenneth N. Gormly
Attorney at Law, PLLC
1107 1/2 Tacoma Ave S
Tacoma, WA 98402
253-274-0500

SAMPLE LETTER FROM A NEUROLOGIST

To Whom It May Concern,

Jane Smith was initially seen by me on August 25, 2003. She was initially thought to have a cervical disk problem; however, she eventually developed other symptoms suggesting a more widespread problem in the nervous system and with clinical findings, supported by an MRI scan, a diagnosis of multiple sclerosis was made. Over the last two years, she has continued to have symptoms suggesting active multiple sclerosis including difficulty walking, and sensory and visual symptoms. Associated with this is a feeling of fatigue and exacerbation of symptoms by heat. All of these create impairments, which significantly limit her physical ability to perform any substantial gainful work.

Mrs. Smith now carries a diagnosis of chronic progressive multiple sclerosis, and it is very likely that this impairment can be expected to last for a continuous period over the years.

Multiple sclerosis in itself is not expected to result in her death; however, it is a disabling disease and it is likely that there will be continued disability.

I have reviewed the Basic Work Capabilities Checklist and Activities of Daily Living questionnaires, and I agree with the outline given by Mrs. Smith.

Again, it is my best judgment that Mrs. Smith's illness of chronic progressive multiple sclerosis limits her from gainful employment at this time and certainly into the foreseeable future.

Sincerely,

[Doctor's Name]

SAMPLE LETTER FROM AN EMPLOYER

To Whom It May Concern,

During the 93–94 school year, Jane Smith became ill and was diagnosed as having multiple sclerosis. The onset of the disease was sudden and dramatic. Jane's physical mobility decreased rapidly along with her physical stamina. It was quickly apparent that accommodations would have to be made in order to assist Jane in continuing her teaching duties.

Accommodations had to be made in three areas: Facilities, Duties, and Work Day.

Facilities:

1. Hinge adjustments were made to the doors to the staff area, office area, classrooms, and restrooms so that Jane could open them.

2. The parking lot was restriped to assist Jane in parking closer to the entryway that was closest to her classroom.

3. The room assignment configuration was adjusted to ensure that Jane's classroom was close to an entryway. This meant that the normal grouping of grade level students could not occur.

Duties:

1. Jane was released from all staff, committee, and student supervision obligations.

2. Other staff were assigned to accompany and supervise Jane's students during field trips.

Work Day:

1. Jane's full-time contract was adjusted so that she could teach half-time.

2. A substitute was hired to teach the other half of her contract. Some weeks went according to schedule with Jane teaching half-days.

3. As the disease continued to be unpredictable in its manifestations, we adjusted the substitute's role so that Jane could be released whenever she needed to be. As time progressed, Jane needed more rest; thus, the substitute was asked to be available for either half or full day work whenever needed.

If you need further information, please call at the number above.

Sincerely,

[Employer's Name]

The Daily Activity Questionnaire

The DDS will often ask for more information in order to make a determination of (legal) disability. That's right, they want even more information to supplement the very thorough application form you already submitted. They may send you a Daily Activity Questionnaire, Activities of Daily Living and Socialization form, Work History Report, and/or a Fatigue Questionnaire.

The bad news: Another #%#*%$&* Form! Another %$*& Deadline!

The good news: Another opportunity to emphasize the total burden of your illness and how it prohibits you from working full-time at ANYTHING. By this time you've probably thought, "Rats! I should have mentioned _____ in that initial application!" Well, here's your chance to work it in.

More good news: You haven't been denied yet!

You can help DDS estimate your "residual functional capacity" for work by describing the activities you perform at home, away from home, in social settings, and your hobbies. Detail the types of assistance you need to complete various tasks. Also include descriptions of activities you used to do, but are no longer able to perform. Tell why and how you do any of those activities differently now. If the categories below are not included on the particular form sent to you, put the information into the "Is there anything else you would like us to know?" item.

The numbered questions below are suggested from various SSA forms and other questionnaires. The follow-up questions are designed to coax out relevant details. If you are stimulated to remember something that doesn't have a corresponding question, just find an appropriate place to insert your information.

You may draft paragraphs for each section or for each question. I suggest organizing the information into the following categories:

- Self-care

- Personal business

- Home care

- Typical month

- Hobbies and recreation

- Social activities

SELF-CARE

1. Do you need help taking care of your personal needs/grooming?

   - What kind of help are you given and how often?

   - Describe any personal tasks that you must do differently now.

   - What personal grooming tasks take longer now? How much longer?

2 Describe and give examples of any of the following activities that give you difficulty.

   - Bathing/showering

   - Grooming (shaving, applying make-up, styling hair)

   - Dressing

   - Eating

   - Brushing your teeth

   - Toileting

   - Taking medication

     - How often do you experience difficulty with each?

     - Tell if the difficulty is mild, moderate, or severe.

     - Describe any procedural adaptations or assistive devices you use to perform these activities.

   - Sleeping

     - How many hours do you sleep?

     - Do you require rest periods during the day?

     - How long is a typical nap?

     - Where do you nap? (bed, couch, chair, recliner)

     - What happens if you're unable to nap?

PERSONAL BUSINESS

1. Describe any difficulties you have with the following tasks. Detail any changes you have made in the way you accomplish each one compared to the way you did when your health was not an issue.

    - Using the phone

    - Shopping

        - Do you do ANY shopping? What kind, how often?

        - If you require assistance, describe the help you receive.

        - Are your trips of shorter duration than before?

        - Are you able to shop at malls?

        - Do you shop online or by catalog because of your condition?

2. Getting places

    - How far from your home is the nearest place you go on a regular basis? How far is the farthest place you go to on a regular basis?

    - How do you usually travel when you go out? (drive, walk, ride the bus, take a cab, ride with friends)

    - Do you need help to go out? What kind of help?

    - Do you drive?

    - Do you use manual, automatic, or hand controls on your vehicle?

    - If you no longer drive, tell when and why you stopped.

    - Are there any restrictions on your driver's license?

    - How far can you drive at one time?

    - Do you have a disabled placard?

    - Do you have difficulty traveling by bus, boat, train, or plane?

        - What happens to you when you travel this way?

3. Making appointments on time

4. Maintaining financial records

    - Who handles the money for your household? If it is you, list the responsibilities.

HOME CARE

1. Where do you live and with whom?

    ■   Do you care for others in your household? (children, adults, pets)

    ■   Describe what you do for them and how these activities affect you.

2. Describe what things you do on a typical day and how these activities make you feel.

    ■   How much time do you spend in each activity?

    ■   How long can you continue until you have to stop?

    ■   What stops you?

3. Describe any stairs inside/outside your home.

    ■   How often do you use these stairs each day?

    ■   Describe the way you must climb them.

4. Tell what/why you have changed anything in your home (removed carpet, mounted grab bars, rearranged furniture, etc.) to accommodate your condition.

5. Do you prepare your own meals?

    ■   How many days a month do you prepare breakfast/lunch/dinner?

    ■   For how many people?

    ■   Describe the extent of preparation, cooking, serving, cleanup you do for the meals you prepare.

    ■   What help do others provide?

    ■   Do you use shortcuts like frozen or packaged meal "kits," purchased bakery items, salads in a bag, etc.?

    ■   Do you regularly cook extra amounts to freeze/reheat on your bad days?

    ■   Do you need to take rest breaks or sit down while you chop veggies or do other kitchen prep?

6. Do you do the housework where you live? Do you do yard work?

    ■   What types and how often do you do these chores and/or do you need assistance in doing them?

    ■   What chores do other people do around your home?

- What home-care tasks don't get done because of your health?

- Are there tasks you used to do but can no longer perform?

- What makes these tasks too difficult for you now?

TYPICAL MONTH

1. In a typical month, how many *good, fair,* and *bad* days do you experience?

   - Give examples of how *fair* and *bad* days differ from *good* days.

2. What causes you to function worse on *fair* and *bad* days?

3. How many days a month does your health keep you at home?

4. Are you functioning better, worse, or about the same as a year ago?

HOBBIES AND RECREATION

1. Describe any hobbies or recreation you now enjoy.

   - How often do you engage in these activities?

   - How much time do you spend at each activity in a typical month?

2. Describe any hobbies or recreational activities you once enjoyed but are no longer able to enjoy because of your health.

   - What keeps you from pursuing these activities now?

3. Do you watch TV? Listen to the radio? Read?

   - How many hours a day?

   - What types of things do you watch/listen to/read?

4. Do you go out to visit friends or relatives?

   - How often do you go out?

   - How long at a time?

   - Where do you get together with others?

   - What do you do when you are together?

SOCIAL ACTIVITIES

1. Are you active in clubs or other social activities? Describe them.

   ■ How often do you do these activities?

   ■ What do you do?

   ■ How long do you spend in these activities?

   ■ What type of places do you go to participate?

2. Tell about your social contacts.

   ■ Tell how each has changed because of the MS in relation to frequency of participation, duration of events, etc.

   ■ List any activities you have given up because of your MS and tell why you no longer pursue them.

   ■ Has MS changed the way you entertain at home?

Document the Impact of Your Multiple Sclerosis with Diary and Worksheets

DIARY TIPS

A diary with rating scales (such as the attached samples), although subjective, does allow you to quantify your experiences. Using a rating scale saves time when recording and assessing data and it takes little effort compared to a narrative description. Adapt the following evaluation system to document and quantify your daily experiences.

The important thing is to START NOW! It is not necessary to write diary entries. Keep a calendar by your bed and write good, bad, or okay on the date before you nod off to sleep. Even smiley faces will do. Get your spouse to write something for you if you are unable to lift the pencil, but put down something on paper every day. At the end of the week, you'll have some useful information and you'll have even better data at the end of the month.

Tip: At your first opportunity, take a moment to jot down what constitutes a good day for you, and list at least three characteristics. Repeat the process for "okay" and "bad" days. Combine this information with the following scale to create a daily log that's meaningful to you. In the long run, this will ensure consistency in your evaluations.

Example:

Minimum attributes of a GOOD day:

1. No severe pain

2. Adequate energy

3. Ability to focus attention

Next, describe a typical good day. Tell what you are able to do, for how long, and with how much or how little assistance. You'll soon be able to review any given day at a glance.

RATING SCALES

Activity Level:

> 1 = slug-like (in bed most of day)
>
> 2 = coping (seated activity only)
>
> 3 = typical (limited walking, standing)
>
> 4 = zippy (able to walk up stairs)
>
> 5 = vigorous (vacuuming, gardening, etc.)

Pace:

> Spurt = 5 to 30 minutes of activity before resting
>
> Sustained = 30 or more minutes of activity before resting

Energy Level:

> 1 = necessities only
>
> 2 = low
>
> 3 = moderate
>
> 4 = high
>
> 5 = normal (how you used to feel before MS)

Pains/Symptoms: Severity:

> 1 = buzzing; fidgets

2 = pins and needles; bug bites

3 = electric shocks; voodoo pins; bee stings

4 = thunderbolts; knifepoint

5 = stun gun; psycho knives

Pain/Symptoms: Frequency:

1 = single occurrence

2 = a few episodes with several hours between occurrences

3 = several episodes occurring in streaks; clusters

4 = many episodes occurring frequently

5 = symptom is present constantly

> **Tip:**   Creating daily schedules for "good" and "bad" days will work too.

S   M   T   W   Th   F   S

Date: _____

Activities/Energy	*Pains/Symptoms*
Activity #1	**Symptom 1:**
Description: _____	Location: _____
Time: Morning Afternoon Evening	Time: Morning Afternoon Evening Night
Level: 1 2 3 4 5	Severity: 1 2 3 4 5
Pace: Spurt Sustained	Frequency: 1 2 3 4 5
Time Spent: _____	**Symptom 2:**
Activity #2	Location: _____
Description: _____	Time: Morning Afternoon Evening Night
Time: Morning Afternoon Evening	Severity: 1 2 3 4 5
Level: 1 2 3 4 5	Frequency: 1 2 3 4 5
Pace: Spurt Sustained	**Symptom 3:**
Time Spent: _____	Location: _____
Activity #3	Time: Morning Afternoon Evening Night
Description: _____	Severity: 1 2 3 4 5

Time: Morning Afternoon Evening

Level: 1 2 3 4 5

Pace: Spurt Sustained

Time Spent: _____

Energy

Morning: 1 2 3 4 5

Afternoon: 1 2 3 4 5

Evening: 1 2 3 4 5

Sleep/Rest

Nap/Rest

Length: _____

Time: Morning Afternoon Evening

Sleep

Total Hours: _____

Times Awakened: _____

Reasons Awakened: _____

Notes:

Frequency: 1 2 3 4 5

Symptom 4:

Location: _____

Time: Morning Afternoon Evening Night

Severity: 1 2 3 4 5

Frequency: 1 2 3 4 5

Medications and Dosage

☐ 1.@ _____ A.M./P.M.

☐ 2.@ _____ A.M./P.M.

☐ 3.@ _____ A.M./P.M.

☐ 4.@ _____ A.M./P.M.

☐ 5.@ _____ A.M./P.M.

☐ 6.@ _____ A.M./P.M.

Weather

Temperature: _____

Conditions: _____

USING THE WORKSHEETS

The following worksheets can be helpful in documenting the impact of fatigue on your daily activities, work functioning, and other nonfatigue symptoms as they also impact your daily activities, and your job functioning. Simply copy as many other symptom worksheets as you need.

MS FATIGUE WORKSHEET

Information about your fatigue and how it affects daily activity

Describe your MS-related fatigue: ■   Tell how it differs from "normal" tired or sleep feelings. ■   Give a graphic example of how it feels.
Do you take any medication for your fatigue?
Does your fatigue follow any discernable pattern?
What level of activity produces your fatigue?
Do you ever become fatigued to the point of incapacity? ■   How often? ■   How long does that extreme condition typically last?
How many hours of sleep do you need each night?
How often and how long do you need to nap or rest?
Is your fatigue affected by heat or any other conditions?
Do your other symptoms become aggravated when you are fatigued? ■   Which ones?
To what degree does fatigue restrict your normal daily activities? (Use specific numbers/amounts when possible.)
List anything your doctor has told you to do (such as rehabilitation or physical therapy) or not to do (restrictions in environments or reduced hours). **Note**: *Give the doctor's name and the date you were told to cut back or otherwise alter your activities.*

MS FATIGUE WORKSHEET (CONTINUED)

Information about how fatigue deeps you from working

Which of these basic physical activities did this symptom limit (check all that apply):				
☐ Sitting	☐ Standing	☐ Walking	☐ Lifting	☐ Carrying
☐ Handling	☐ Pushing	☐ Pulling	☐ Reaching	☐ Climbing
☐ Stooping	☐ Crouching	☐ Seeing	☐ Hearing	☐ Speaking

How often were you absent from your job during the last six months you worked because of fatigue?

How did fatigue get in your way?

What did fatigue keep you from doing?

What were you unable to do as much as before?

What were you unable to do as well as before?

What did you have to do differently?

How many times a day/week/month did fatigue interfere with your work?

MS SYMPTOM WORKSHEET

Information about this symptom

Is this symptom present most of the time or does it come and go?
How often does this symptom occur (frequency)?
How long does this symptom last (duration)?
What happens to your body?
Where does this symptom affect you (body location)?
How does this symptom feel? (Give a graphic example.)
Does a particular activity or environment make this symptom occur?
In what way does this symptom limit your normal activities?
To what degree does this symptom restrict your normal daily activities? (Use specific numbers/amounts when possible.)
List anything your doctor has told you to do (such as rehabilitation or physical therapy) or not to do (restrictions in environments or reduced hours). **Note:** *Give the doctor's name and the date you were told to cut back or otherwise alter your activities.*

MS SYMPTOM WORKSHEET (CONTINUED)

Information about how this symptom keeps you from working:

Which of these basic physical activities did this symptom limit (check all that apply):

☐ Sitting ☐ Standing ☐ Walking ☐ Lifting ☐ Carrying

☐ Handling ☐ Pushing ☐ Pulling ☐ Reaching ☐ Climbing

☐ Stooping ☐ Crouching ☐ Seeing ☐ Hearing ☐ Speaking

How did this symptom get in your way?

What did it keep you from doing?

What were you not able to do as much as before?

What were you unable to do as well as before?

What did you have to do differently?

How many times a day/week/month did this symptom interfere with your work?

Resources

Accommodation Resources: Work and Independent Living

ABLEDATA (www.abledata.com)

Rehabilitation Engineering and Assistive Technology Society of North America (www.resna.org)

West Virginia University's Job Accommodation Network (JAN) (www.jan.wvu.edu)

Advocacy

British Columbia Ombudsman (www.ombudsman.bc.ca)

Alcohol Screening

Join Together, as part of Demand Treatment initiative (www.alcoholscreening.org)

Alternative Medicine Information

Rocky Mountain MS Center Complementary and Alternative Medicine Program (www.ms-cam.org/CAMbanner.htm)

Attorneys/Social Security

National Organization of Social Security Claimants' Representatives (www.nosscr.org)

General Information/Services

Consortium of Multiple Sclerosis Centers (www.mscare.org). *International Journal of MS Care* on Web site.

Multiple Sclerosis Association of America (www.msaa.com)

Multiple Sclerosis Foundation (www.msfocus.org)

Multiple Sclerosis Society of Canada (www.mssociety.ca)

National Multiple Sclerosis Society (www.nmss.org)

University of Washington Multiple Sclerosis Research and Training Center (www.msrrtc.washington.edu)

Legal Rights

Department of Justice (www.usdoj.gov)

Medicaid

State Medicaid agencies (www.cms.hhs.gov)

Personalized MS Information/Chat Room Options

MSWatch (www.mswatch.com/community). Maintained by pharmaceutical company.

Relaxation Strategies

Mind/Body Medical Institute (www.mbmi.org)

Social Security Information

Social Security Administration (www.ssa.gov/work)

References

Agency for Healthcare Research and Quality. 2002. S-Adenosyl-L-Methionine for Depression, Osteoarthritis, and Liver Disease. Summary, Evidence Report/Technology Assessment: No. 64. AHRQ Publication No. 02-E033, Rockville, MD., August 22.

Allen, D. 2001. *Getting Things Done: The Art of Stress-Free Productivity*. New York: Viking.

Archbold, P., and B. Stewart. 1990. Mutuality and preparedness as predictors of caregiver role strain. *Research in Nursing & Health* 13(6):375-384.

Archbold, P., B. Stewart, and M. Hornbrook. 2001. *Family Care Inventory*. Portland, OR: School of Nursing, Oregon Health & Science University.

Basso, M., M. Beason-Hazen, J. Lynn, R. Rammohan, and R. Bornstein. 1996. Screening for cognitive dysfunction in multiple sclerosis. *Archives of Neurology* 53:980-984.

Beatty, W., R. Paul, B. Wilbanks, K. Hames, C. Clanco, and D. Goodkin. 1995. Identifying multiple sclerosis patients with mild or global cognitive impairment using the Screening Examination for Cognitive Impairment (SEFCI). *Neurology* 45:718-723.

Bourne, E. 2005. *The Anxiety and Phobia Workbook*. 4th ed. Oakland, CA: New Harbinger Publications.

Bowling, A. 2001. *Alternative Medicine and Multiple Sclerosis*. New York: Demos.

Bowling, A., R. Ibrahim, and R. Stewart. 2000. Alternative medicine and multiple sclerosis: An objective review from an American perspective. *International Journal of MS Care* 2:14-21.

Bowling, A., and T. Stewart. 2003. Current complementary and alternative therapies of multiple sclerosis. *Current Treatment Options in Neurology* 5:55-68.

Brinkman, M. J., G. D. Henty, S. K. Wilson, Jr., R. Delk II, G. A. Denny, M. Young, et al. 2005. A survey of patients with inflatable penile prostheses for satisfaction. *Journal of Urology* 174:253-257.

Burns, D. D. 1999. *Feeling Good.* New York: W. Morrow.

Chwastiak, L., D. Ehde, L. E. Gibbons, M. Sullivan, J. D. Bowen, and G. H. Kraft. 2002. Depressive symptoms and severity of illness in multiple sclerosis: Epidemeological study in a large community sample. *American Journal of Psychiatry* 159:1862-1868.

Clemmons, D., R. Fraser, G. Rosenbaum, A. Getter, and E. Johnson. 2004. An abbreviated neuropsychological battery in multiple sclerosis (MS) vocational rehabilitation: Findings and implications. *Rehabilitation Psychology* 49:100-105.

Confavreux, C., S. Veekusic, T. Moreau, and P. Adeleine. 2000. Relapses and progression of disability in multiple sclerosis. *New England Journal of Medicine* 343:1430-1438.

Davis, M., E. Eschelman, and M. McKay. 2000. *The Relaxation and Stress Reduction Workbook.* 5th ed. Oakland, CA: New Harbinger Publications.

Dello Buono M., O. Urciuoli, and D. Deleo. 1998. Quality of life and longevity: A study of centenarians. *Age and Ageing* 27:207-216.

Ehde, D., and C. Bombardier. 2005. Depression in persons with multiple sclerosis. *Physical Medicine and Rehabilitation Clinics of North America* 16:437-448.

Ehde, D., L. Osborne, and M. Jensen. 2005. Chronic pain in persons with multiple sclerosis. *Physical Medicine and Rehabilitation Clinics of North America* 16:503-510.

Eisenberg, D. M., R. B. Davis, S. L. Ettner, S. Appel, S. Wilkey, M. Van Rompay, et al. 1998. Trends in alternative medicine use in the United States, 1990-1997: Results of a follow-up national survey. *JAMA* 280:1569-1575.

Fraser, R., B. McMahon, and R. Danczyk-Hawley. 2003. Progression on disability benefits: A perspective on multiple sclerosis. *Journal of Vocational Rehabilitation* 19:173-179.

Good D., D. Bower, and R. Einsporn. 1995. Social support: Gender differences in multiple sclerosis spousal caregivers. *Journal of Neuroscience Nursing* 27:305-311.

Goodin, D., E. Frohman, G. Garmany, Jr., J. Halper, W. Likosky, F. Lublin, et al. 2002. Disease modifying therapies in multiple sclerosis: Report of the Therapeutics and Technology Assessment Subcommittee of the American Academy of Neurology and the MS Council for Clinical Practice Guidelines. *Neurology* 58:169-178.

Greenberger, D., and C. Padesky. 1995. *Mind over Mood.* New York: Guilford Publishing.

Guarnaccio, J., and J. Booss. 2005. An overview of multiple sclerosis. In *Multiple Sclerosis: A Self-Care Guide to Wellness.* Edited by J. Halper and N. J. Holland. New York: Demos.

Halper, J. 2005. General health issues. In *Multiple Sclerosis: A Self-Care Guide to Wellness.* Edited by J. Halper and N. J. Holland. New York: Demos.

Hensiek, A., R. Roxburgh, and A. Compston. 2003. Genetics of multiple sclerosis. In *Multiple Sclerosis 2.* Edited by W. McDonald and J. Noseworthy, 75-92. Philadelphia: Butterworth Heinemann.

Jacobs, L., D. Cookfair, R. Rudick, R. Herndon, J. Richaert, A. Salazar, et al. 1996. Intra-muscular Interferon Beta-1a for disease progression in relapsing remitting multiple sclerosis. The Multiple Sclerosis Collaborative Research Group (MSCRG). *Annals of Neurology* 39:285-294.

Johnson, K., K. Yorkston, E. Klasner, C. Kuehn, and D. Amtmann. 2004. The cost and benefits of employment: A qualitative study of experiences of individuals with multiple sclerosis. *Archives of Physical Medicine and Rehabilitation* 85(2):201-209.

Kinkel, R., K. Cenway, L. Copperman, S. Forwell, C. Hugos, D. Mohr, et al. 1998. Fatigue and multiple sclerosis: Evidence-based management strategies for fatigue in multiple sclerosis. Washington, DC: Multiple Sclerosis Council for Clerical Practice Guidelines, Paralyzed Veterans of America.

Kraft, G., and J. Cui. 2004. Multiple sclerosis. In *Physical Medicine and Rehabilitation: Principles and Practice*. Edited by J. Delina, B. Gans, and N. Walsh, 1753-1769. Philadelphia: J. B. Lippincott.

Kraft, G., J. Freal, J. Coryell, C. Hanan, and N. Chitnisn. 1981. Multiple sclerosis: Early prognostic guidelines. *Archives of Physical Medicine and Rehabilitation* 62:54-58.

Kraft, G. and R. Taylor. 1998. Preface. Physical Medicine and Rehabilitation. *Clinics of North America*. Aug., pp xi-xii.

Krupp, L., L. Alvanex, N. LaRocca, and L. Scheenberg. 1988. Fatigue in multiple sclerosis. *Archives of Neurology* 45:435-437.

Kurtzke, J. 2005. Epidemiology and etiology of multiple sclerosis. *Physical Medicine and Rehabilitation Clinics of North America* 16:327-350.

Kurtzke, J., and M. Wallin. 2000. Epidemiology. In *Multiple Sclerosis: Diagnosis, Medical Management, and Rehabilitation*. Edited by J. Berkes and K. Johnson. New York: Demos.

LaRocca, N. 2005. Personal Communication, National Multiple Sclerosis Society. May 5.

LaRocca, N., and H. Hall. 1990. Multiple sclerosis program: A model for neuropsychiatric disorders. *New Directions for Mental Health Services* 45:49-64.

LaRocca, N., and R. Kalb. 2005. Addressing cognitive problems. In *Multiple Sclerosis: A Self-Care Guide to Wellness*. Edited by J. Halper and N. J. Holland. New York: Demos.

LaRocca, N., R. Kalb, L. Scheinberg, and P. Kendell. 1985. Factors associated with unemployment of patients with multiple sclerosis. *Journal of Chronic Disease* 38:203-210.

Laumann, E. D., and C. Rosen 1999. Sexual dysfunction in the United States: Prevalence and predictors. JAMA 281:537-544.

Law, N., and B. Noyes. 2005. Work, family, and community participation. In *Multiple Sclerosis: A Self-Care Guide to Wellness*. Edited by J. Halper and N. J. Holland. New York: Demos.

Loehr, J., and T. Schwartz. 2003. *The Power of Full Engagement: Managing Energy, Not Time, Is the Key to High Performance and Personal Renewal*. New York: Free Press.

Lublin, F., M. Baier, and G. Cutter. 2003. Effect of relapses on the development of residual deficit in multiple sclerosis. *Neurology* 61:1528-1532.

MacAllister, W., and L. Krupp. 2005. Multiple sclerosis–related fatigue. *Physical Medicine and Rehabilitation Clinics of North America* 16:483-502.

McCurdy, D. B. 1998. Personhood, spirituality, and hope in the care of human beings with dementia. *Journal of Clinical Ethics* 9;81-91.

McDonald W., A. Compston, G. Edan, D. Goodkin, H. Hartung, F. Lublin, et al. 2001. Recommended diagnostic criteria for multiple sclerosis: Guidelines from the international panel on the diagnosis of multiple sclerosis. *Annals of Neurology* 50(1):121-127.

McKay, M., M. Davis, and P. Fanning. 1997. *Thoughts & Feelings: Taking Control of Your Moods and Your Life.* Oakland, CA: New Harbinger Publications.

McKeon, L. P., and A. P. Porter-Armstrong. 2004. Caregives of people with multiple sclerosis: Experiences of support. *Multiple Sclerosis* 10:219-230.

McNulty, K., H. Livneh, and L. Wilson. 2004. Perceived uncertainty, spiritual well-being, and psycholsocial adaptation in individual with MS. *Rehabilitation Psychology* 49:91-99.

Mohr, D. C., C. Classen, and M. Borrera, Jr. 2004. The relationship between social support, depression, and treatment for depression in people with multiple sclerosis. *Psychological Medicine* 34:533-541.

National Multiple Sclerosis Society. 2003. *Multiple Sclerosis Information Sourcebook.* http://www.national mssociety.org/ sourcebook.asp.

National Multiple Sclerosis Society. 2005. Disease management consensus statement. New York.

Padma, N., W. Hellstrom, F. Kaiser, R. Labasky, T. Lue, W. Nolten, et al. 1997. Treatment of men with erectile dysfunction with transurethal alprostadil: medicated urethral system for erection (MUSE) study group. *New England Journal of Medicine* 336:1-7.

Pakenham, K. 1999. Adjustment to multiple sclerosis: Application of a stress and coping model. *Health Psychology* 18:383-392.

Pittock S., W. Mayr, R. McClelland, N. Jorgensen, S. Weigand, J. Noseworthy, et al. 2004. Disability profile of MS did not change over 10 years in a population-based prevalence cohort. *Neurology* 62(4):601-606.

Prochaska, J., J. Norcross, and C. DiClemente. 1994. *Changing for Good: A Revolutionary Six-Stage Program for Overcoming Bad Habits and Moving Your Life Positively Forward.* New York: Avon Books.

Rao, S. 1995. Neuropsychology of multiple sclerosis. *Current Opinion in Neurology* 8(3):216-220.

Rao, S., T. Hammeke, M. McQuillen, B. Khatri, and D. Lloyd. 1984. Memory disturbance in chronic progressive multiple sclerosis. *Archives of Neurology* 41(June):625-631.

Rao, S., G. Leo, L. Bernardin, and F. Unverzagt. 1991. Cognitive dysfunction in multiple sclerosis. I. Frequency, patterns, and prediction. *Neurology* 41:686-691.

Rao, S., G. Leo, L. Ellington, T. Nauertz, L. Bernardin, and F. Unverzagt. 1991. Cognitive dysfunction in multiple sclerosis. II. Impact on employment and social functioning. *Neurology* 41:692-696.

Roessler, R., and J. Gottcent. 1994. The work experience survey: A reasonable accommodation/career development strategy. *Journal of Applied Rehabilitation Counseling* 25:16-21.

Rosenberg, S. 2005. Clinical Overview of Multiple Sclerosis. Symposium presentation at the Annual Conference of the National Consortium of Multiple Sclerosis Centers. Orlando, FL, May, June 4.

Rothwell, P., Z. McDowell, C. Wong, and P. Dorman. 1997. Doctors and patients don't agree: Cross sectional study of patients' and doctors' perceptions and assessments of disability on multiple sclerosis. *British Medical Journal* 314:1580.

Rumrill, P., Jr. 1996. *Employment Issues and Multiple Sclerosis.* New York: Demos.

Ryan, D. 2000. *Job Search Handbook for People with Disabilities.* Indianapolis, IN: JIST.

Sanders, A. S., F. W. Foley, N. B. LaRocca, and V. Zemon. 2000. The multiple sclerosis intimacy and sexuality questionnaire-19 [MSISQ=19]. *Sexuality and Disability* 18(1):3-26.

Shelton, R. C., M. B. Keller, M. Gellenburg, D. L. Dunner, R. Hirschfield, M. E. Those, et al. 2001. Effectiveness of St. John's wort in major depression: A randomized controlled trail. *JAMA* 285:1978-1986.

Solomon, A. 2001. *The Noonday Demon: An Atlas of Depression*. New York: Scribner's.

Stryon, W. 1990. *Darkness Visible: A Memoir of Madness*. New York: Random House.

Stuifbergen, A., and S. Roberts. 1997. Health promotion practices of women with multiple sclerosis. *Archives of Physical Medicine and Rehabilitation* 78:53-59.

Sullivan, G. 2005. M5 as a spiritual journey. *Inside* 23:58-63.

Yorkston, K., K. Johnson, E. R. Klasner, D. Amtmann, C. Kuehn, and B. Dudgeon. 2003. Getting the work done: A qualitative study of experiences of individuals with multiple sclerosis. *Disability and Rehabilitation* 25:369-379.

Zorzon, M., R. Zivadinov, A. Bocco, L. M. Bragadin, R. Moretti, L. Bonfiglio, et al. 1999. Sexual dysfunction in multiple sclerosis: A case controlled study. I. Frequency and comparison of groups. *Multiple Sclerosis* 5:418-427.

Robert T. Fraser, Ph.D., is a licensed counseling and rehabilitation psychologist and professor of neurology, neurological surgery, and \rehabilitation medicine at the University of Washington. He specializes in specializes in vocational rehabilitation assessment and counseling for people with MS and is one of the original faculty of the University of Washington MS Rehabilitation Research and Training Center.

George H. Kraft, MD, MS, is the director of the Western MS Center. He specializes in the rehabilitation of multiple sclerosis.

Dawn M. Ehde, Ph.D., is a psychologist and associate professor in the Department of Rehabilitation Medicine at the University of Washington. She specializes in the treatment of st in pain and depression in persons with management and works to help people with multiple sclerosis and other disabilities. improve their physical functioning through a wide variety of rehabilitation techniques.

Kurt L. Johnson, Ph.D., is a professor in the Department of Rehabilitation Medicine at the University of Washington. He specializes in psychosocial aspects of disability, disability and employment, assistive technology, and disability policy

Some Other
New Harbinger Titles

The Cyclothymia Workbook, Item 383X, $18.95

The Matrix Repatterning Program for Pain Relief, Item 3910, $18.95

Transforming Stress, Item 397X, $10.95

Eating Mindfully, Item 3503, $13.95

Living with RSDS, Item 3554 $16.95

The Ten Hidden Barriers to Weight Loss, Item 3244 $11.95

The Sjogren's Syndrome Survival Guide, Item 3562 $15.95

Stop Feeling Tired, Item 3139 $14.95

Responsible Drinking, Item 2949 $18.95

The Mitral Valve Prolapse/Dysautonomia Survival Guide, Item 3031 $14.95

Stop Worrying Abour Your Health, Item 285X $14.95

The Vulvodynia Survival Guide, Item 2914 $15.95

The Multifidus Back Pain Solution, Item 2787 $12.95

Move Your Body, Tone Your Mood, Item 2752 $17.95

The Chronic Illness Workbook, Item 2647 $16.95

Coping with Crohn's Disease, Item 2655 $15.95

The Woman's Book of Sleep, Item 2493 $14.95

The Trigger Point Therapy Workbook, Item 2507 $19.95

Fibromyalgia and Chronic Myofascial Pain Syndrome, second edition, Item 2388 $19.95

Kill the Craving, Item 237X $18.95

Rosacea, Item 2248 $13.95

Thinking Pregnant, Item 2302 $13.95

Shy Bladder Syndrome, Item 2272 $13.95

Help for Hairpullers, Item 2329 $13.95

Coping with Chronic Fatigue Syndrome, Item 0199 $13.95

The Stop Smoking Workbook, Item 0377 $17.95

Multiple Chemical Sensitivity, Item 173X $16.95

Breaking the Bonds of Irritable Bowel Syndrome, Item 1888 $14.95

Parkinson's Disease and the Art of Moving, Item 1837 $16.95

The Addiction Workbook, Item 0431 $18.95

The Interstitial Cystitis Survival Guide, Item 2108 $15.95

Call **toll free, 1-800-748-6273,** or log on to our online bookstore at **www.newharbinger.com** to order. Have your Visa or Mastercard number ready. Or send a check for the titles you want to New Harbinger Publications, Inc., 5674 Shattuck Ave., Oakland, CA 94609. Include $4.50 for the first book and 75¢ for each additional book, to cover shipping and handling. (California residents please include appropriate sales tax.) Allow two to five weeks for delivery.

Prices subject to change without notice.